W9-AHG-846

YOGA | FOR INFLEXIBLE PEOPLE

Thunder Bay Press
An imprint of Printers Row Publishing Group
10350 Barnes Canyon Road, Suite 100, San Diego, CA 92121
www.thunderbaybooks.com • mail@thunderbaybooks.com

Copyright © 2020 Max & Liz Lowenstein
Cover image: Fizkes/Shutterstock, Inc

All rights reserved. No part of this book may be reproduced,
distributed, or transmitted in any form or by any means, including
photocopying, recording, or other electronic or mechanical methods,
without the prior written permission of the publisher, except in the
case of brief quotations embodied in critical reviews and certain other
noncommercial uses permitted by copyright law.

Printers Row Publishing Group is a division of Readerlink Distribution
Services, LLC. Thunder Bay Press is a registered trademark of
Readerlink Distribution Services, LLC.

Correspondence regarding the content of this book should be
sent to Thunder Bay Press, Editorial Department, at the above
address. Author, illustration, and rights inquiries should be addressed
to Welbeck Publishing Group • www.welbeckpublishing.com

Publisher: Peter Norton • Associate Publisher: Ana Parker
Acquisitions Editor: Kathryn C. Dalby
Editor: JoAnn Padgett

Produced by Welbeck Publishing Group

ISBN: 978-1-64517-492-9

Printed in Slovenia

24 23 22 21 20   1 2 3 4 5

Please note
The authors and publisher cannot accept any responsibility for
misadventure or injury resulting from the practice or application
of any of the principles and techniques set out in this book. Not
all exercise is suitable for everyone. It is recommended that you
consult your doctor or healthcare professional before embarking
on this or any other exercise program. Do not force or strain your
body to achieve any of the postures. This book is not intended as
a substitute for medical attention, diagnosis, or treatment; if you
are in any doubt about any aspect of your condition, please refer
to a medical professional.

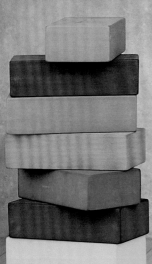

YOGA | FOR INFLEXIBLE PEOPLE

MAX & LIZ LOWENSTEIN

THUNDER BAY
P·R·E·S·S
San Diego, California

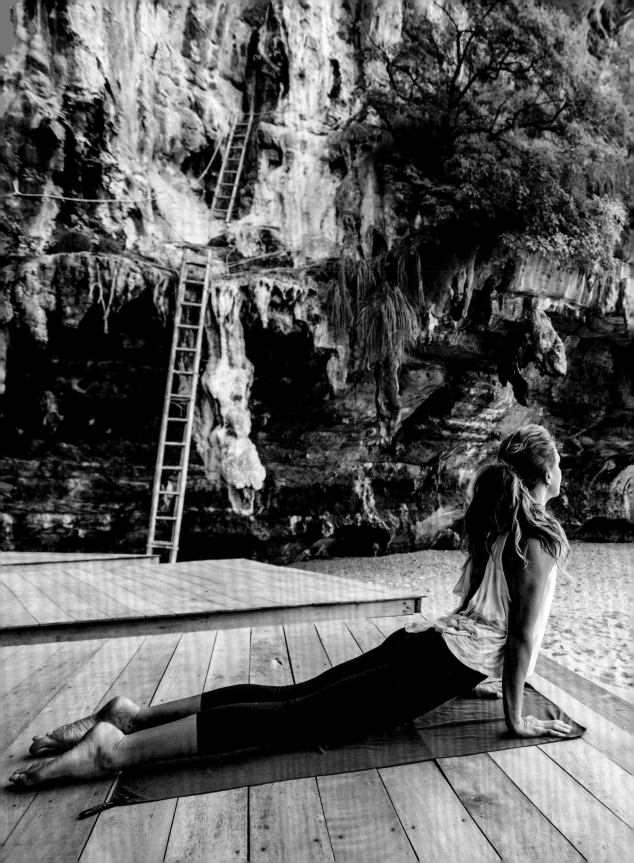

CONTENTS

INTRODUCTION

When I was a teenager, my mother insisted I had to come home early three times a week from basketball to practice yoga. I hated it. I thought it was both foolish and embarrassing. However, after just a few months, I started to see the benefits and actually began to look forward to it.

During college I found that yoga was something girls were into and I practiced on and off until I had a steady girlfriend, but then I abandoned it. Just before I graduated, when I was at the peak of my inflexibility (in both a mental and physical sense), my mother sent me a video of a yogini doing some powerful arm balances. This was when my life changed forever: I saw someone who could be both impressively strong and flexible. I was inspired.

After college, I began to do yoga many times a day for the physical benefits it provided, but I suffered a number of injuries. This coincided with the darkest time of my life. I began to explore yoga more deeply, and this was when I came to think of it as a way of life, rather than just a physical practice.

I decided to train as a yoga teacher and fell in love with AcroYoga. I now travel all over the world with my beautiful wife teaching workshops, retreats, and festivals, with an emphasis on anatomy and hand balancing. Yoga has taken me from a stressed, anxious, reactive, and aggressive place to one of calmness, where I can choose my response to whatever life throws at me.

Max

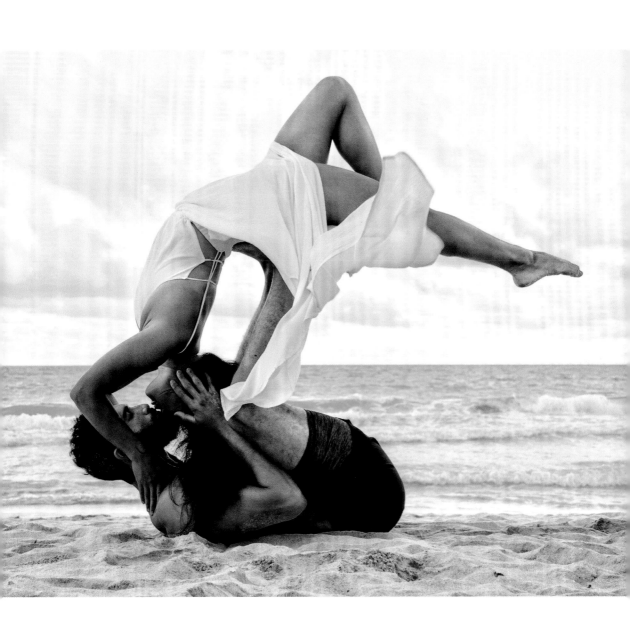

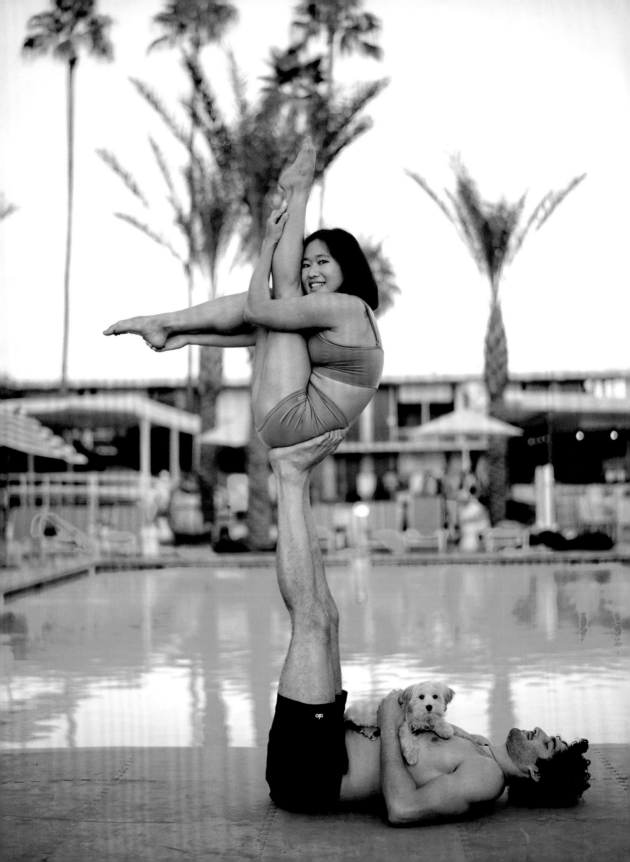

I was eighteen when I found yoga—or rather, when yoga found me. I was a competitive swimmer in high school but decided to abandon the sport in college. To try to keep in shape I found some yoga sessions online and practiced in my room with a cheap yoga mat—I was too scared to go to an actual class.

Yoga began as a workout, trying to "master" each move, treating it as my next goal. Through each movement, each class, each savasana, each year, each life transition, I learned to breathe through difficult poses and situations; to let go with more grace; to flow with more ease; and, above all, to connect with my whole self on the mat, so that I could connect with others off the mat.

Liz

"Our mission is to help the global community gain ease and flexibility in both body and mind. We aim to aid people along their journeys, every step of the way. Whether you're an aspiring yogi, looking for a recovery method or supplementing your training routines, you have come to the right place."

We created this book to show the progressions from beginner to advanced variations of poses, accessible to anyone, anywhere on their yoga journey. You don't have to be the most flexible person to begin with; you can start wherever you are and honor your body throughout the process. Remember, flexibility is both in the body and in the mind. Thoughts become words, words become actions—everything is connected and is vibration in another form.

We started our Instagram account, @inflexibleyogis, to create a community of people who could support one another when starting their yoga/flexibility journeys. We want you to savor and cherish every moment, as well as valuing every step you make along the way! The pictures we share are designed to inspire and educate. On the following pages are images and inspirational quotes from our devoted followers that show how regular and committed practice means progress!

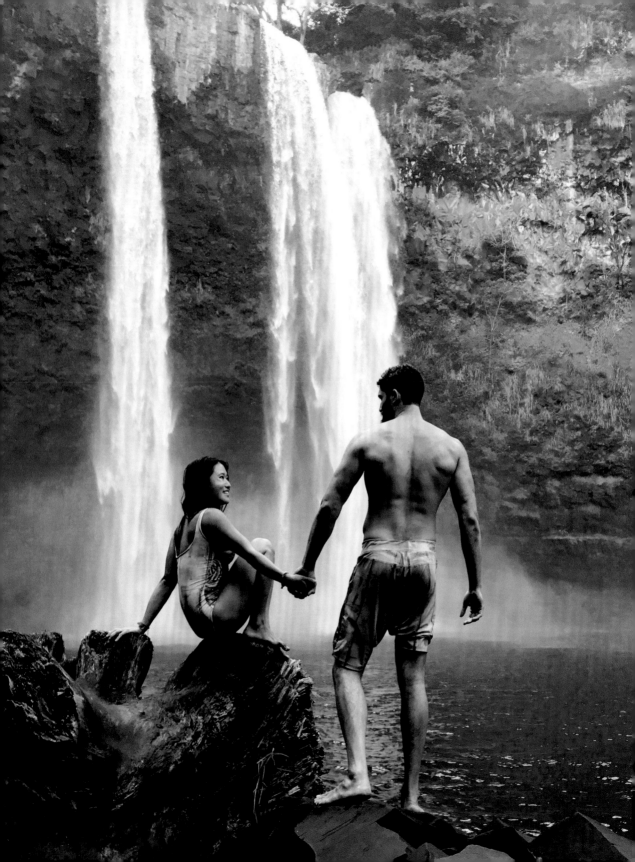

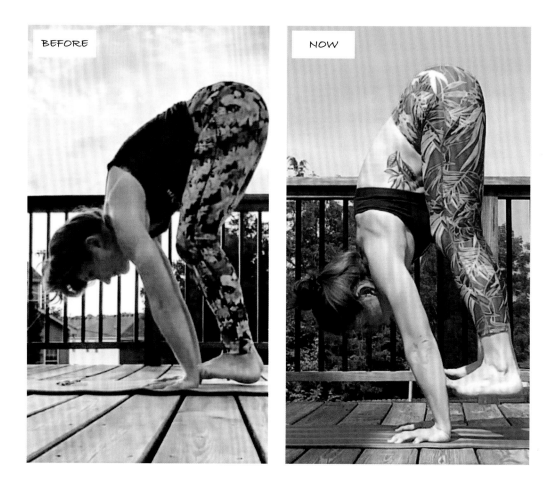

BEFORE

NOW

"Ten years after heart surgery, I became a certified power yoga teacher at the age of thirty-nine. If I can build a handstand and inversion practice, anyone can! I believe yoga is a portal to learn more about yourself, and a fountain of youth, keeping the body and mind open and strong."

Reb Gibson

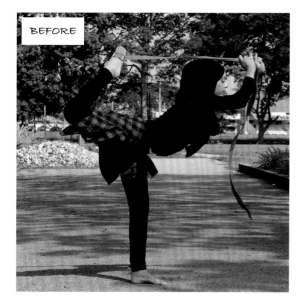

BEFORE

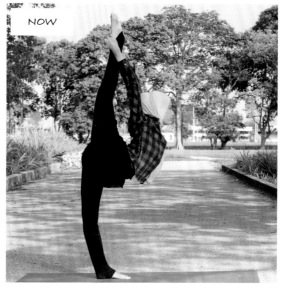

NOW

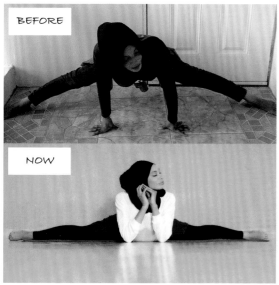

BEFORE

NOW

"I discovered Yoga in a very dark place in my life. I was thirty-three years old. Prior to that, I had no flexibility background but I was determined for this to change. I put all my energy into my daily practice, which made me flexible. I see yoga as the cure that healed my mind, body, and soul. I am still learning as yoga is a continual process of discovery."

Shaeeda Sween

"I've never had self-esteem. I was a shy girl, unsure and afraid of standing in the light. I used to be good at nothing. For a long time, I hated myself; I hated everything about myself: body, mind, everything. And even though, I became stronger and stronger facing difficulties everyday, my self-esteem was always low. I felt good at nothing. Then one day, after days and days of looking at other yogis, I decided to start yoga. I got better and better. I got so much better that one day something HUGE happened: I felt I was GOOD at something. All of a sudden, I opened my eyes and realized how good I was. Not because of the fancy poses I managed to do, but because of the effort I put into my practice.

I practiced, and practiced, and practiced. And one day, all of a sudden, looking at one of my yoga pictures, I realized that it was not just a picture, it was so much more. I could see the practice behind the picture, the effort, the perseverance and the commitment. And I felt good at something for the first time in my life. For all of you thinking about starting something new like yoga...do it. No matter what that is, just do it. Step out of your comfort zone and do it. I promise it's going to be the best thing you've ever done."

Miss Erica

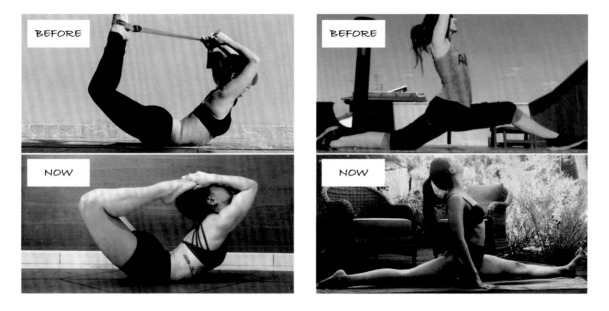

BEFORE

NOW

BEFORE

NOW

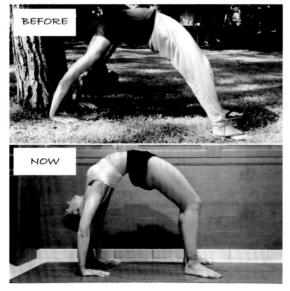

BEFORE

NOW

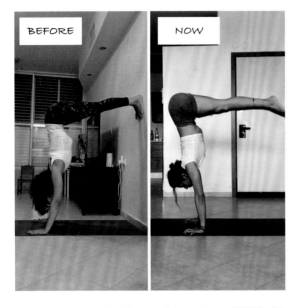

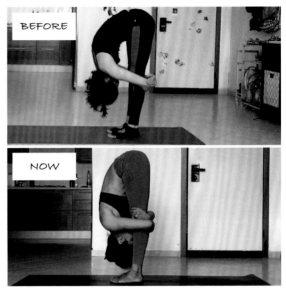

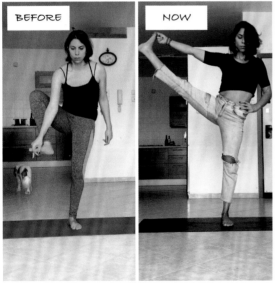

"A handstand was something I didn't even dream of because I had such weak arms and shoulders, and just the thought of falling kept me from trying. During my yoga journey, I've come to realize that my body can do more than I ever gave it credit for. For three years, I have been practicing. Now I can stand on my hands, and that feels pretty amazing."

Yoga Vered

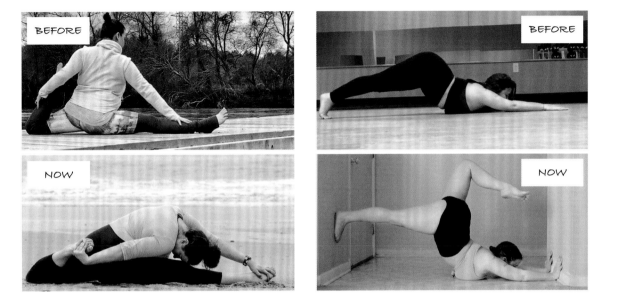

"Yoga asks you to be humble within both success and failure. To press forward when you feel defeated. To be consistent and patient when you feel frustrated. Within the progression of the physical practice you become humble, consistent, and patient with yourself."

Joe Ray

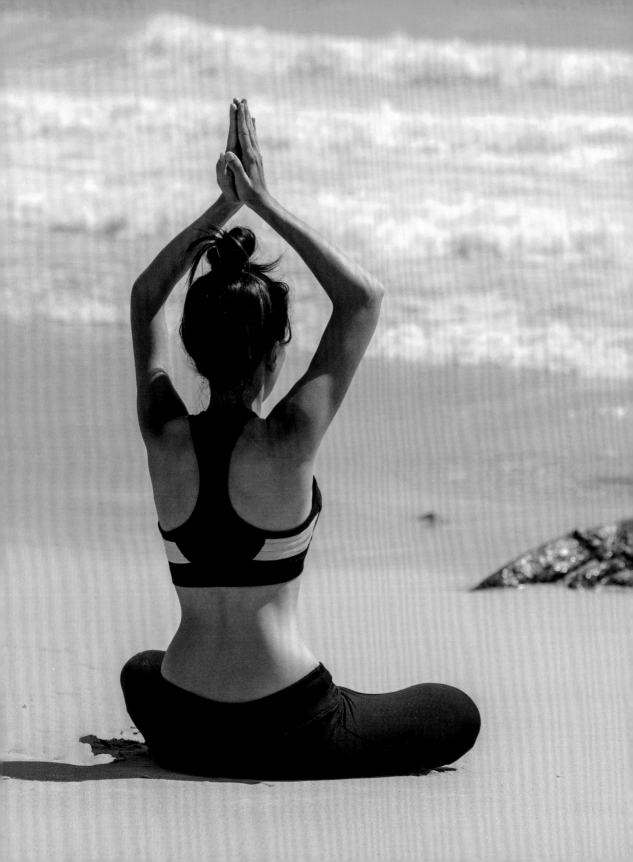

1

GETTING STARTED

You can begin your yoga/flexibility journey anytime and
anywhere! You don't need to be a certain size, shape, or
age—this is about coming into your power and connecting
to your body and movement. In this opening section we will
explore flexibility, what it is and why it is important. We move
on to discuss how today's lifestyle can impact our spine health
and physical well-being and what we can do to counteract this
process. Yoga practice requires some basic equipment, so we
will look at what you need and how this can help your practice
and enable you to progress. We examine some key postures
that are used as reference points for many of the poses
covered in the book, and for warming up, which is essential
to loosen up the spine, neck, wrists, and other joints before
beginning your practice. Finally, we offer three breathing
exercises that calm the mind.

WHAT IS FLEXIBILITY?

Flexibility begins in the mind. The first step is to create your own vision of what you want for your body, and with practice and perseverance the rest will follow. The journey toward flexibility is something to be valued and enjoyed.

In terms of physiology, flexibility is the range of motion in a joint or a group of joints, or the extent to which a group of muscles can be stretched. Your range of motion or level of flexibility can vary greatly for different parts of your body. Developing your flexibility can help to counteract the demands of daily life, protect against injury, and promote your general well-being.

Yoga and flexibility go hand in hand. Yoga is a discipline that includes breath control and specific postures that involve stretching and meditation. Combined with mindfulness and using your breath, yoga can improve your level of flexibility, increase the range of motion throughout your body, and make you feel longer and leaner.

Benefits of flexibility

1. Corrects posture and improves balance—increasing flexibility helps spine alignment and strength.

2. Improves your state of mind—work on flexibility brings about feelings of relaxation.

3. Increases range of motion—a well-stretched muscle more easily achieves its full range.

4. Improves circulation—increased blood flow to soft tissues promotes faster healing.

Relieves pain and muscle soreness—when muscles are looser and less tense, you feel fewer aches and pains.

 Improves movement performance—across a range of different activities.

7 Prevents injuries—once strength increases, more physical stress can be placed on the body.

SPINE HEALTH

The health of your spine is essential to the rest of your body. The spine houses the central nervous system along which is carried every impulse that is sent to or from the brain. Most of us spend a great deal of time with our heads down and our shoulders hunched—be it at work over a computer or on the bus or the train over our phone or tablet.

Over time this lack of movement in our spines causes the ligaments between the vertebrae to harden and the muscles to tighten. In turn this hinders the transmission of messages along the central nervous system, which can cause decreased sensation, pain, disease, slower recovery, impaired sleep, slower reflexes, and poor performance. However, with regular exercise and the correct maintenance, the health of the spine can be restored with a range of benefits that are both mental and physical.

PROGRESSING TO GREATER FLEXIBILITY

The book is structured so that it targets all the components of flexibility. Each chapter builds on the one before to open up the different parts of the body and prepare for the next sections.

The postures in this book progress in three stages—beginner, intermediate, and advanced. How long it takes to move on to each stage depends on the individual. Everyone is different and people hold tension in different ways. Here are some general tips to progression:

- Be aware of how you feel during each stage and hold each posture as long as it feels comfortable.

- Breathe into the body, allowing all parts to open and release.

- Mild discomfort is fine but if you experience a sharp, stabbing feeling in a particular area then you are moving too quickly and this may lead to injury.

- Practicing the postures regularly over time will aid your progression.

Good spine health means:

1 Improved cognition

2 Mood enhancement

3 Regular sleep patterns

4 Better memory

5 Better performance

6 Increased work capacity

7 Improved hand-eye coordination

8 Faster recovery

EQUIPMENT

Yoga requires minimal equipment—the practice is about you and your body. However, there are a few items that are helpful, particularly when starting out. The first of these is a mat to provide comfort, safety, and support. You can also use props such as blocks and straps to help you in your poses; these act as an extension of your body when you are working toward a posture. Whether you are aiming to touch your feet or the floor, or to clasp your hands behind your back, yoga props are amazing at aligning our bodies, and should be seen as tools, not crutches. The correct clothing is also important: form-fitting clothing with a good stretch is essential so you can check your position but feel comfortable and supported at all times.

MATS

Mats provide a cushion for the knees and other joints while practicing yoga and working on flexibility. They also prevent your hands and feet from slipping and mark out your own particular space on the floor.

- Help to keep your body warm and maintain your energy.

- Prevent your hands and feet from slipping.

- Provide support for joints.

- Help define your space when working in a group.

BLOCKS

Think of a block as an extension of yourself. This is a prop that will help you reach your fullest extension. Don't forget that blocks can also be used on a low or high setting, depending on the level at which you are working. This will help you to progress through the different stages of each pose.

- Can be used at a setting that is most suitable for you.

- Help you to progress with flexibility.

- Assist in reaching your maximum extension.

- Help you to stay in poses for longer.

YOGA STRAPS

Straps can be used as extensions of limbs and also to support and lengthen different parts of the body in stretches and holds. They can be helpful in maintaining correct alignment and are especially beneficial if you have tight hamstrings and shoulders.

- Provide support for the body during poses.

- Help you to progress with flexibility.

- Assist in maintaining correct alignment.

- Helpful for those with tight shoulders and hamstrings.

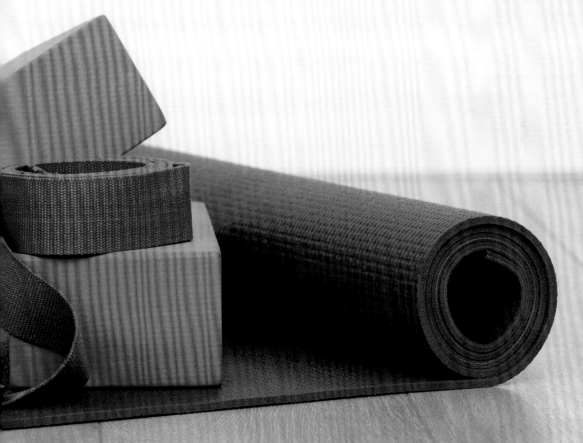

KEY POSTURES

A starting position is essential before beginning any yoga practice. Poses typically begin from standing, a seated position, or on your hands and knees. The three key postures described here give a solid foundation for each of these starting points, as well as providing a transition between poses.

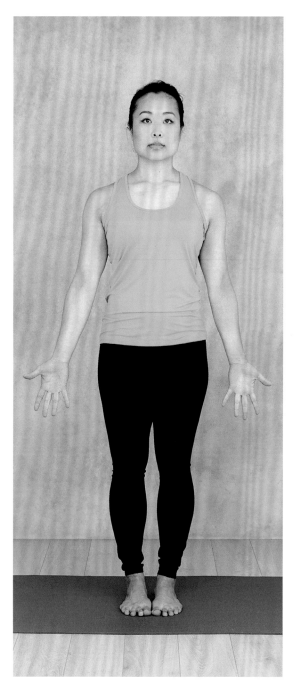

MOUNTAIN POSE

The foundation of all standing poses, mountain pose improves posture and strengthens the whole body.

1 Stand with your toes touching and your heels slightly apart so that the outer edges of your feet are parallel.

2 Engage your thighs and lift your kneecaps.

3 Draw your tailbone down and pull your belly inward and upward.

4 Draw your shoulder blades down your spine.

5 Stand with your arms by your sides and your palms facing forward.

6 Pull your collarbones away from one another.

7 Keep your head neutral.

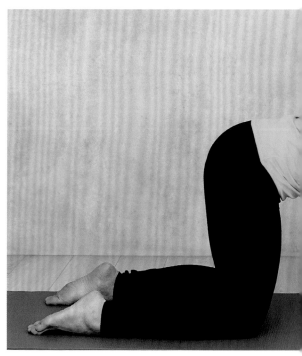

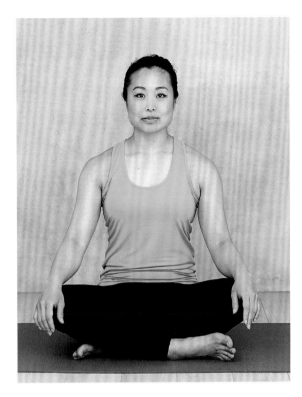

EASY SEATED POSE

This pose calms the brain, prepares the body for meditation, strengthens the back, and stretches the hips, knees, and ankles. You can place a blanket under your sit bones if you need more padding; sit with your back to a wall for more support. Alternatively, you can sit on a block to lift your hips and lengthen your spine.

1   Sit on the floor (or on a block or blanket).

2   Cross your shins over one another with your feet underneath the opposite knee. You can place blocks under your knees for support.

3   Draw your shoulder blades down your spine, and keep your spine long and straight.

4   Keep your head neutral.

5   Place your hands on your knees with your palms facing down or with your thumb and index finger touching.

6   Hold for 5–10 breaths, and then repeat with your legs crossed the other way.

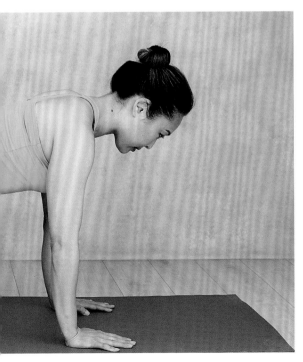

TABLE TOP

This pose provides a transition to other poses such as downward-facing dog (*see pages 126–127*), puppy dog pose (*see pages 56–57*), and plank (*see pages 110–111*).

1   Start on your hands and knees with your arms shoulder-width apart and your shoulders stacked over your wrists.

2   Stack your hips over your knees.

3   Engage your core.

4   Keep your head neutral.

WARMING UP

Although yoga may appear to be "gentle" exercise, practice involves challenging and stretching the muscles and working the joints, so including a warm-up before you begin is extremely important. Loosening the muscles and joints helps to eliminate stiffness and maintain the correct posture during poses, and will also help to prevent injury.

1 Begin in a comfortable seated or standing position with your eyes closed and take several deep breaths in and out through your nose.

2 Fill up your lungs on an inhale and push all the air out on the exhale.

3 Warming up the mind is equally as important as warming up the body; clear your mind and set an intention.

4 Articulate your joints: move your joints in circles slowly in both directions, starting with the neck, followed by the shoulders, arms, elbows, wrists, fingers, hips, knees, ankles, and toes.

CAT/COW

The cat and cow poses warm up and lubricate the spine to prepare for backbends. The cat and cow stretch the back of the torso and neck while strengthening the core and abdominal organs. Coordinating movement with breath relieves stress and calms the mind.

1 **Cow** Begin with a neutral spine in table-top position; inhale, drop your belly and arch your spine; draw the crown of your head and your tailbone up.

2 Cat Exhale, round your spine and tuck your chin into your chest, drawing your shoulder blades away from one another.

3 Start with 10–20 slow rounds, alternating cat and cow poses.

NECK STRETCHES

These exercises stretch the muscles along the length of the spine and the shoulders and also release the trapezius muscles.

1 Stand with your legs hip-width apart and tuck your chin into your chest.

2 With your left hand tilt your head and bring your left ear down to your left shoulder.

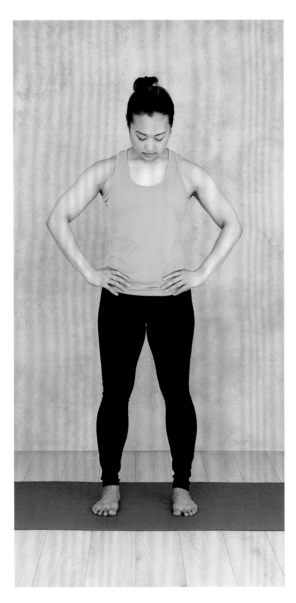

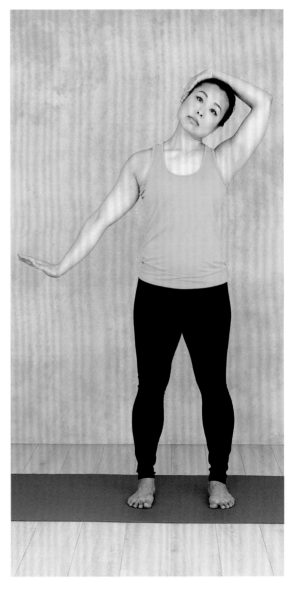

3 Place your hands on your hips, extend your neck, and look up to the sky.

4 Rotate your head, clockwise or counterclockwise, taking your right ear to your right shoulder. Go slowly, taking care of your neck.

5 Make 5–10 rotations and then change direction.

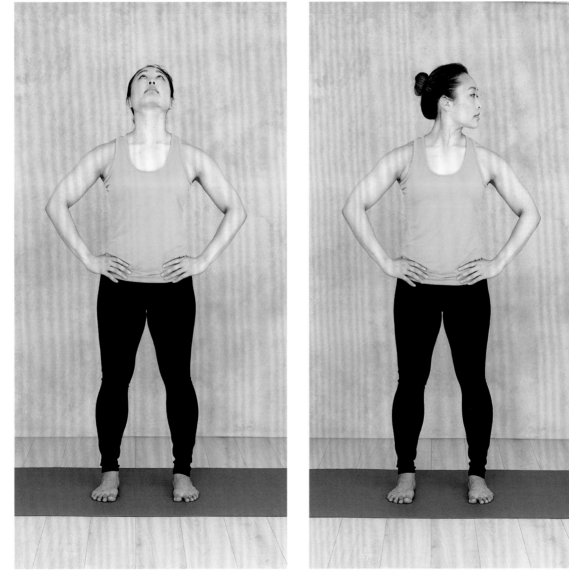

SIDE STRETCHES

Side bends provide balance to your whole body, lengthening the abs, hips, and thigh muscles while improving flexibility in the spine.

1 Start by kneeling or standing in mountain pose (*see page 26*).

2 Grab your right wrist with your left hand; inhale to lengthen your spine, and on the exhale lean to the left, stretching the right side of the body.

3 Come back to center on the next inhale and change sides on the exhale.

4 To go a little deeper, drop one arm down to your side as the other arm reaches up and overhead.

5 Hold and breathe.

6 Change sides on the exhale.

WRIST STRETCHES

Wrist injuries are common in yoga hand balances so warm up your wrists thoroughly before practicing any movement that requires you to put weight on your hands. These exercises will stretch your wrists while strengthening the muscles in your hands and forearms, which in turn will protect your joints.

1 Begin in table-top position with your shoulders stacked over your wrists and your hips stacked over your knees (*see page 27*).

2 Lift the heels of your palms and then slowly bring them down. Keep your arms straight.

3 Repeat 10–20 times.

1 Place your hands under your shoulders with your palms down. Rotate your arms outward until your fingers are facing toward you—or as far as you can go with your arms straight.

2 Lean back and then push yourself forward with your arms straight.

3 Repeat 10–20 times.

1 Place your hands under your shoulders with your palms up. Rotate your arms so that your elbow creases are facing forward.

2 Lean back and then push yourself forward with your arms straight.

3 Repeat 10–20 times.

1 Come onto the backs of your hands making fists and bring your knuckles together.

2 From this position, lower and raise your elbows.

3 Repeat 10–20 times.

A modification that can be made for all of these wrist stretches is to move your knees closer to your hands so that less pressure is placed on the wrists.

BREATHWORK

Breathwork comprises breathing exercises to improve mental, physical, and spiritual health. Yoga breathing exercises ("pranayama" in Sanskrit) are an important part of developing a yoga practice. During breathwork we oxygenate our brain by regulating our inhalations and exhalations. By controlling our breath, we calm our minds and bring awareness to the present moment.

UJJAYI BREATHING

Ujjayi means "to conquer" or "to be victorious." This technique is used throughout Ashtanga and Vinyasa yoga practices and involves filling your lungs completely, while slightly contracting your throat and breathing through your nose. It calms the mind and warms the body.

1 Begin in a comfortable, seated position (*see page 27*).

2 Relax your entire body and close your eyes.

3 Inhale and exhale through your mouth.

4 As you continue, on your exhale contract the back of your throat slightly as if you are fogging up a mirror.

5 Begin to maintain a slight constriction of your throat on the inhales so your breath makes a sound like the sea.

6 Once you are comfortable with this breathwork, close your mouth and inhale and exhale through your nose—still constricting the back of your throat.

7 Breathe deeply, letting each inhale fill your lungs and every exhale release the air completely.

8 Gradually link your breath to movement with yoga poses.

LION'S BREATH

This technique reduces stress, anger, and tension. The powerful exhale provides a way to release negative internal energy and can improve self-esteem and produce feelings of empowerment. Always practice lion's breath in a determined way.

1 Lower your jaw, open your mouth wide, and stick out your tongue, pointing it downward.

2 Lift your gaze to the sky.

3 Exhale forcefully with a "Haaaaa" sound, letting the air pass over the back of your throat.

4 Repeat 2–3 times.

DEEP STOMACH BREATHING

This activates the parasympathetic nervous system and helps to relieve stress and anxiety.

1 Breathe deeply into your stomach.

2 Feel your stomach and lower belly expand.

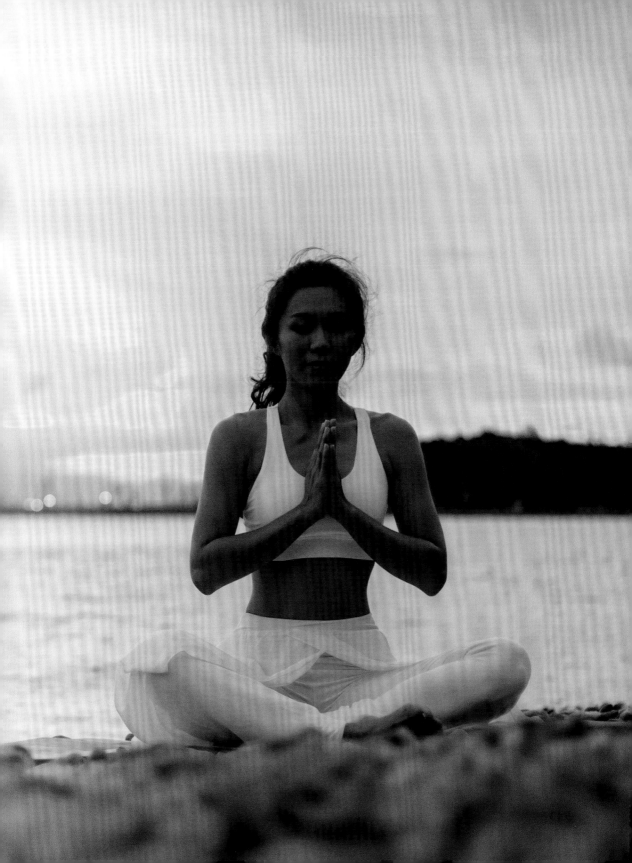

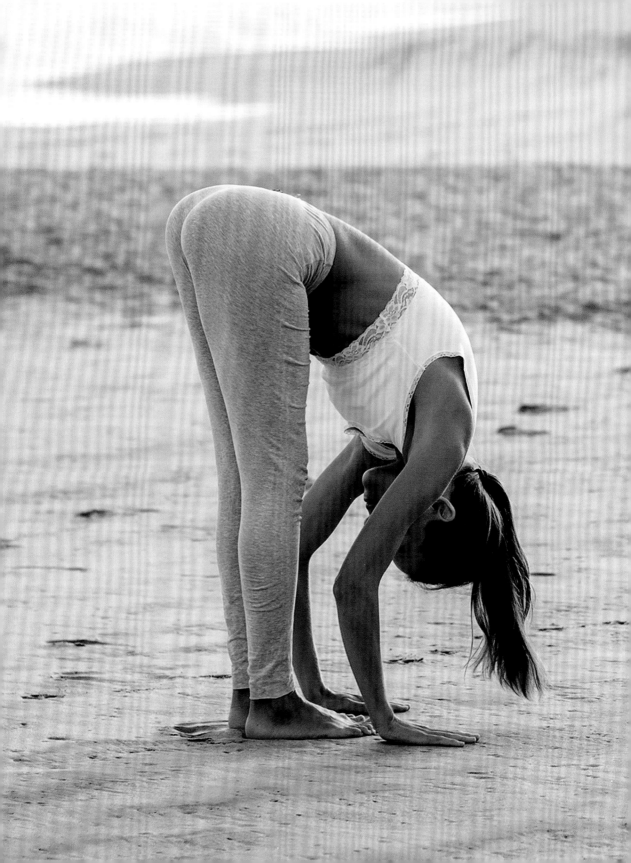

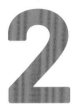

FORWARD FOLDS

These poses involve folding forward at the crease of the hip and stretching all along the back of the body, from your head to your heels. They help to build strength and flexibility in the spine, and tone and stimulate the internal organs, increasing circulation to those in the pelvic region. Forward folds calm the mind, soothe the nervous system, and encourage you to look inward—physically, emotionally, and spiritually—and can help to reduce anxiety, stress, depression, and insomnia. They can be a challenge for some people, especially those with tighter hamstrings or hips, so ensure you use the appropriate modifications and work at the most suitable level for you. Take particular care not to round your back or shoulders, or to overstretch your back muscles. Always move with your breath and don't force yourself into a pose. Surrender to the present, notice the experience, and honor what your body is doing.

STANDING FORWARD FOLD

This posture is appropriate for all levels and provides a highly effective stretch for the spine and hamstrings. Practiced regularly it can relieve back pain and stiffness in the spine. It stimulates the internal organs, improves digestion, and can reduce stress and anxiety.

1	BEGINNER

For those with tighter hamstrings or back injuries, gentler variations of the standing forward fold include bent knees or placing hands on yoga blocks.

1 Take a block and place it at a low or high setting, whichever is the most suitable level for you.

2 From standing, exhale and start to bend forward/fold at the hips down to the floor.

3 Place your hands on the blocks.

4 Draw your kneecaps up toward your hips to engage your quads and protect your knees.

5 Make sure your hips are stacked over your heels.

6 With your back flat, draw your shoulder blades down your back, and your shoulders away from your ears.

7 Inhale to lengthen your spine, exhale to fold a little deeper.

Keep your spine straight

Engage your quads to protect your knees

Keep space between your hands and feet

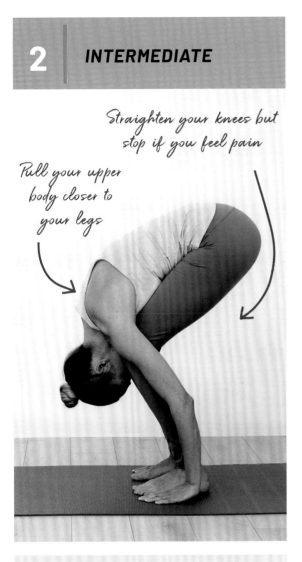

<table>
<tr><td>

2 **INTERMEDIATE**

Straighten your knees but stop if you feel pain

Pull your upper body closer to your legs

</td><td>

3 **ADVANCED**

Pull your chest to your thighs

Keep your legs straight

</td></tr>
</table>

2 INTERMEDIATE

1 Begin as before, this time without blocks.

2 When you exhale, fold forward and rest your hands on the floor next to your feet.

3 Bend your knees as much as you need to allow your chest to touch your thighs; keeping your knees bent protects your lower back.

4 Inhale to lengthen your spine, exhale to fold a little deeper.

3 ADVANCED

1 Begin as before.

2 Exhale, fold forward at the hips, and grab your legs behind your ankles.

3 Make sure your legs are straight, your chest is flat on your thighs, and your back is flat (not rounded).

4 Inhale to lengthen your spine, exhale to fold a little deeper.

PYRAMID POSE

In this intense side stretch, alignment is key. Once a strong base is achieved you can then focus on extending the pose to achieve maximum benefit. This pose can calm the mind, stretch the spine, hips, and hamstrings, and also massage the liver and stomach.

1 | **BEGINNER**

1 Stand with your feet hip-width apart.

2 Step your right foot 3–4ft forward in a scissor stance with both feet rotated outward to 45 degrees.

3 Place a block on either side of your front foot at a low or high setting, whichever is the most suitable level for you.

4 With your hips square, fold down over your thighs and place your hands on the blocks.

5 Pull your belly toward your front thigh but don't round your spine. Draw your ribs in, squeeze your inner thighs, and focus on your front big toe.

6 Push down into the pads of your toes and distribute your weight evenly throughout both feet.

7 Inhale to lengthen your spine, and exhale to fold a little deeper without losing your long, low back. Repeat on the other side.

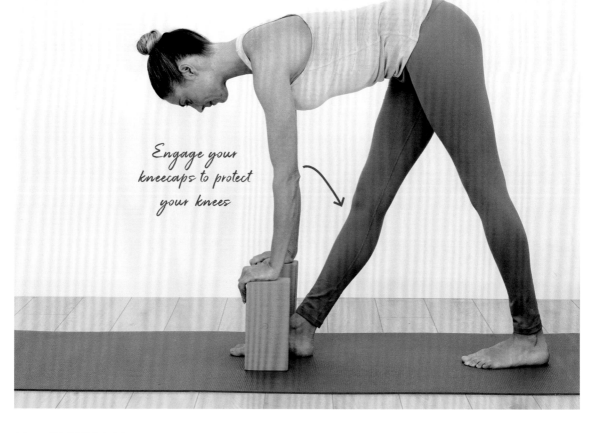

Maintain a flat back

Engage your kneecaps to protect your knees

2 INTERMEDIATE

1. Begin as before, this time without blocks.
2. Place your hands on the floor, shoulder-width apart, in front of your front foot.
3. Bring your belly to your front thigh and fold down over your leg.
4. Inhale to lengthen your spine, and exhale to fold a little deeper. Repeat on the other side.

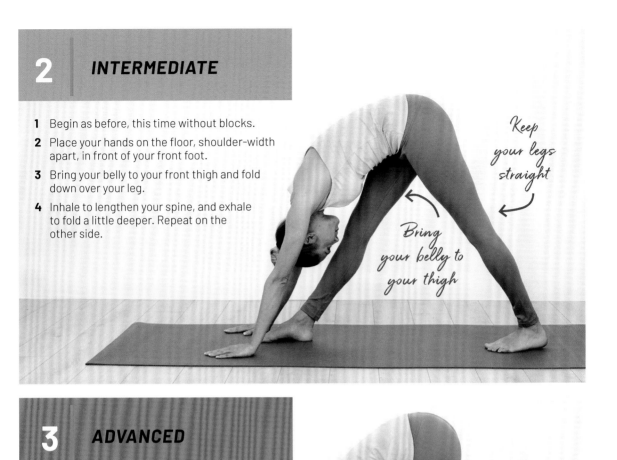

Keep your legs straight

Bring your belly to your thigh

3 ADVANCED

1. Begin as before.
2. Reach your hands behind your front leg and tent your fingers to face the back of the mat.
3. Push down into your fingertips and lift your back leg off the floor, bending your knee and drawing your heel to your glute.
4. Inhale to lengthen your spine, exhale to fold a little deeper. Repeat on the other side.

Glue your belly to your front thigh

Fingers face the back of the mat

STANDING WIDE-LEGGED FORWARD FOLD

This pose works the lower body by stretching the inner thighs, hips, and hamstrings, and it also strengthens and stabilizes the legs. It is known for its revitalizing effects: as the head is lower than the heart, blood flow to the brain is increased.

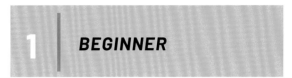

1 | **BEGINNER**

1 Step your feet 3–4ft apart, in line with one another, and your hips square. The outsides of your feet should be parallel with the edges of the mat.

2 Take a block in each hand and place them on the floor underneath your shoulders, at a low or high setting.

3 Exhale and fold forward at the hips with a flat back. Place your hands on the blocks to support your upper body.

4 Inhale to lengthen your spine, then exhale to fold a little deeper.

5 Draw your kneecaps up toward your hips to engage your quads and protect your knees.

6 Ensure your weight is distributed evenly between your feet and across all parts of each foot.

7 To come out of the pose, inhale to halfway up with a flat back, remain still for the exhale, and on the next inhale come all the way up.

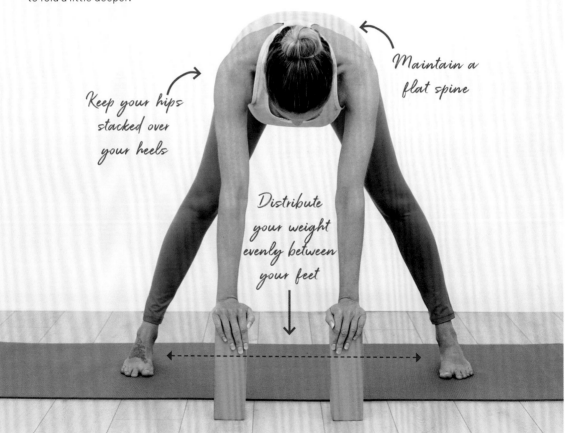

Keep your hips stacked over your heels

Maintain a flat spine

Distribute your weight evenly between your feet

1 Begin as before, this time without blocks.

2 Place your hands on the floor, shoulder-width apart, in line with your feet.

3 Bring the crown of your head to the floor in front of your hands.

4 Walk your hands in to pull your belly closer to your thighs.

5 Inhale to lengthen your spine, then exhale to fold a little deeper.

2 INTERMEDIATE

Squeeze your elbows together

Make sure your fingers are facing forward

1 Begin as before.

2 On the inhale, clasp your hands behind your back.

3 On the exhale, fold down toward the floor with your hands still clasped.

4 Place the crown of your head on the floor and bring your torso in line with your legs. Bring your hands down toward the floor.

3 ADVANCED

Clasp your hands and draw them down to the floor

Keep your torso in line with your legs

SEATED FORWARD FOLD

This pose calms the mind, relieves stress and anxiety, reduces fatigue, and is beneficial for those with high blood pressure. It stimulates the internal organs and improves digestion while providing an effective stretch for the spine, shoulders, and hamstrings.

1	BEGINNER

1 Sit on the floor with your legs straight out in front.

2 Pull the fleshy part of your buttocks away from one another so you are seated just on your sit bones.

3 Press down actively through your heels and flex the feet back, squeezing your legs together.

4 Reach forward with your hands and bend your knees as much as necessary to reach your big toes.

5 Lay your chest on your thighs and keep your spine long.

6 Inhale to lengthen your spine, then exhale to fold down toward your thighs.

Lay your chest on your thighs

Keep your spine long

Flex your feet, squeezing your legs together

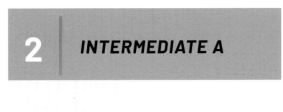

INTERMEDIATE A

1 Begin as before.

2 Wrap the strap around your feet and hold onto the ends.

3 Pull yourself forward with a flat back.

4 Inhale to lengthen your spine, then exhale to fold down toward your feet.

5 When you are ready to go farther, use the strap to progress the pose gradually until you can reach your big toes.

Pull forward toward your feet with a flat back

3 | INTERMEDIATE B

1 Begin as before, this time without the strap.

2 Keep practicing until you can reach your toes. Progress the pose gradually; don't force yourself down into the forward bend by pulling on your feet.

3 Inhale to lengthen your spine, then exhale to fold down farther toward your feet.

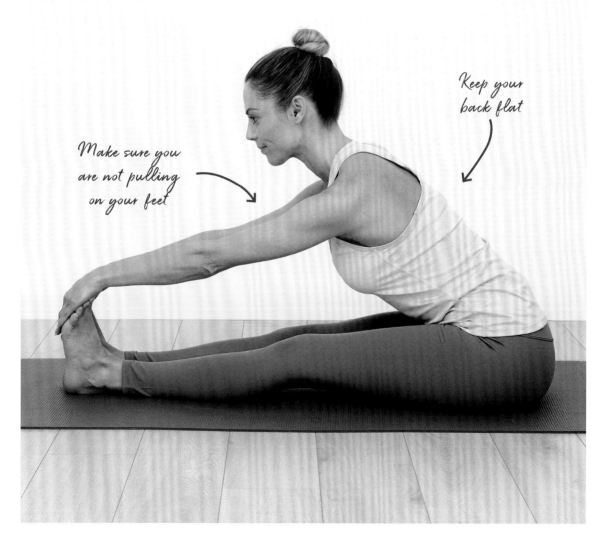

Make sure you are not pulling on your feet

Keep your back flat

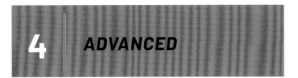

4 ADVANCED

1 Begin as before.

2 Once you are able to hold your toes, work toward bringing your belly to your thighs.

3 Engage your kneecaps, bringing them up toward your hips to protect your knees.

4 Bring your nose down toward your toes and your chin to your shins.

5 Your lower belly should touch your thighs first, followed by your upper belly, your ribs, and finally your head.

6 Bend your elbows to the side as you fold down. Eventually you may be able to stretch your arms out on the floor beyond your feet.

7 Inhale to lengthen your spine, then exhale to fold down farther.

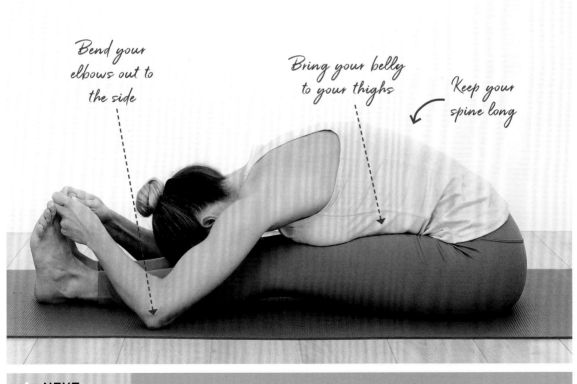

Bend your elbows out to the side

Bring your belly to your thighs

Keep your spine long

NEXT LEVEL

If you can fold all the way forward, try wrapping your hands around your feet, then grab one wrist with the other hand.

HEAD-TO-KNEE FORWARD FOLD

This pose focuses on one leg at a time and provides a twist, stretching the spine, shoulders, hamstrings, and the groin. It is good for the digestion, stimulates the liver and kidneys, and can help to relieve menstrual discomfort.

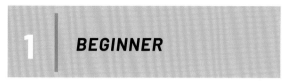

1 | **BEGINNER**

1 Sit on the floor with your legs straight out in front.

2 Bend your left knee and place your heel on your right inner thigh, close to your perineum.

3 Turn your upper body slightly to the right, squaring your torso to your right leg and lining up your belly button with the middle of your right thigh.

4 Hook the strap around your right foot.

5 Hold onto the ends of the strap with both hands and lean forward with a straight back.

6 Inhale to lengthen your spine, then exhale to fold a little deeper.

7 To come out of the pose, inhale and bring your torso back up to a sitting position. Repeat on the other side.

Line up your belly button with the middle of your right thigh

Lean forward with a straight back

2 INTERMEDIATE

1 Begin as before.

2 When you are ready, without using the strap, inhale and reach out with your hands toward your right foot.

3 Exhale and extend forward from the crease of your hips, keeping your back flat.

4 As you fold, bend your elbows out to the sides and lift them away from the floor, keeping your shoulders away from your ears. Repeat on the other side.

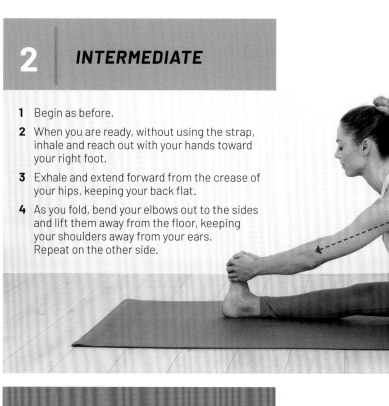

Keep your shoulders down

Bend your elbows to the sides

3 ADVANCED

1 Begin as before.

2 Inhale to lengthen your spine, then exhale to fold down toward your thighs.

3 Your lower belly should touch your thigh first, followed by your head. Take care not to force yourself down into the pose. Repeat on the other side.

Bring your head to your knee

Lower your belly to your thigh

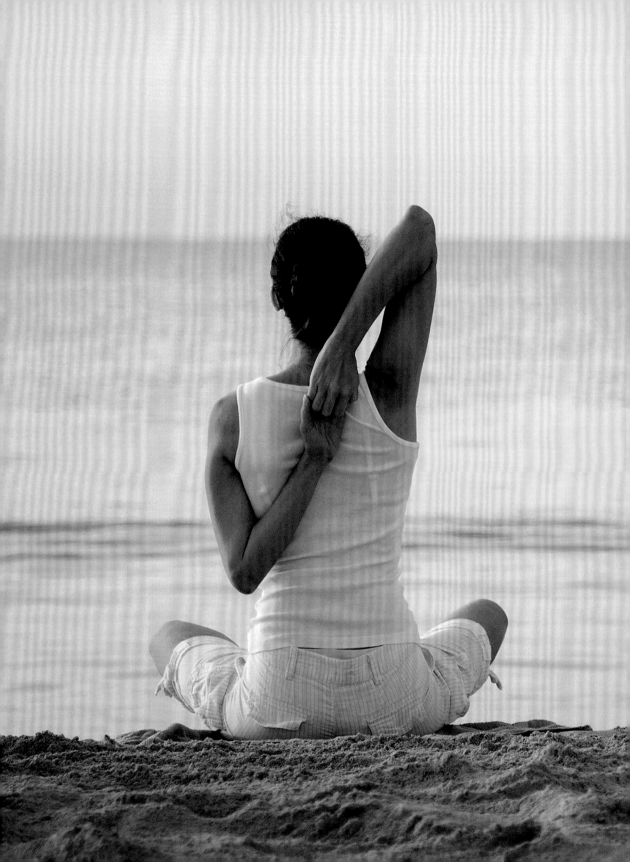

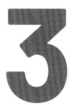

SHOULDER OPENERS

Poor posture can shorten the muscles in the shoulders, neck, and upper back. Yoga in general, and shoulder opener poses in particular, can stretch out and loosen the muscles in these areas, thereby reducing chronic muscle pain and joint discomfort, improving posture, increasing the range of motion, and relieving tension in the head, neck, and shoulders. Yoga poses like shoulder openers activate the heart chakra, which is associated with love, compassion, and security. Occasionally, these poses can produce feelings of slight panic as we tend to store many different emotions in this energetic center, but if you practice regularly, you can truly open your heart.

CHILD'S POSE

Child's pose is a common resting position used at the beginning, middle, or end of a yoga practice and is an excellent opener for the shoulders and spine. It relaxes the muscles at the front of the body while passively stretching the hips, back, thighs, and ankles.

1 Begin on your hands and knees.

2 Spread your knees wide so that your big toes are touching and your glutes are on your heels. If your hips are tight, you can keep your knees and thighs together.

3 Inhale, sit up straight, and lengthen through your spine.

4 Exhale, lean forward, and relax your upper body. Your heart and chest should rest between or on top of your thighs.

5 Place your forehead on the floor with your arms down beside your legs, palms facing toward the sky.

6 To come out of the pose, use your hands to walk your torso to an upright position and sit back on your heels.

Rest your heart and your chest between or on top of your thighs

Relax the tension in your shoulders, arms, and neck

Make sure your big toes are touching

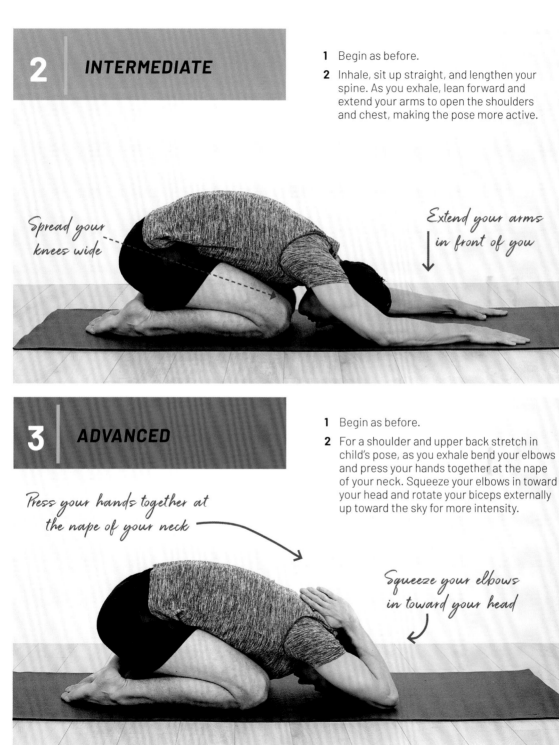

2 | INTERMEDIATE

1 Begin as before.
2 Inhale, sit up straight, and lengthen your spine. As you exhale, lean forward and extend your arms to open the shoulders and chest, making the pose more active.

Spread your knees wide

Extend your arms in front of you

3 | ADVANCED

1 Begin as before.
2 For a shoulder and upper back stretch in child's pose, as you exhale bend your elbows and press your hands together at the nape of your neck. Squeeze your elbows in toward your head and rotate your biceps externally up toward the sky for more intensity.

Press your hands together at the nape of your neck

Squeeze your elbows in toward your head

PUPPY DOG POSE

This pose opens the heart and the shoulders and is a good way to reenergize yourself after a day at work. As well as stretching all parts of the upper body, the down pose also helps to lengthen the spine and relieve stress and tension.

1 Begin in table-top position (*see page 27*).

2 Start to walk your hands forward, making sure your hips stay over your knees.

3 Position two blocks in front of your elbows and place your elbows on the blocks at a low or high setting.

4 Place your palms together above your head. Keep your arms active but relax your head and neck. If your shoulders are tight, your head doesn't need to touch the floor. Breathe into the shoulders on every inhale and exhale.

5 Inhale to lengthen your spine and exhale to sink a little deeper.

6 To come out of the pose, lower your arms and walk your hands back to table-top position.

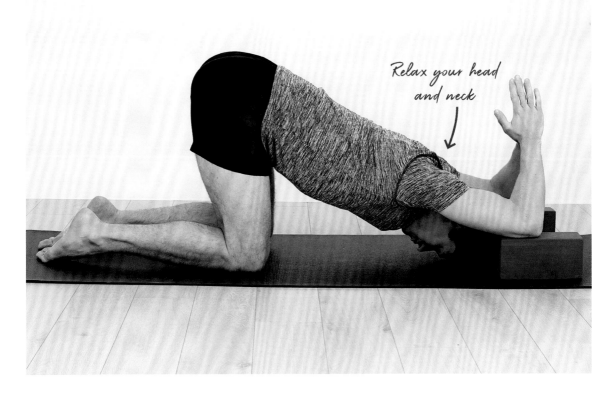

Relax your head and neck

1 Begin as before, this time without blocks.
2 Walk your hands forward, keeping your hips over your knees, until your chin comes into contact with the floor.

3 Inhale to lengthen your spine and exhale to sink a little deeper.
4 To come out of the pose, walk your hands back to return to table-top position.

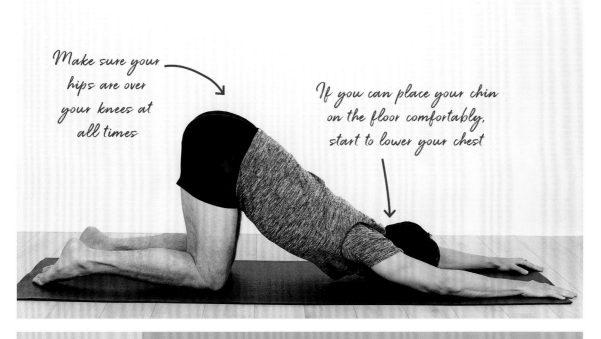

Make sure your hips are over your knees at all times

If you can place your chin on the floor comfortably, start to lower your chest

NEXT LEVEL

Slowly lower your chin and chest so they eventually come down to the floor as your shoulders become more open.

REVERSE PRAYER POSE

As well as opening the chest and loosening the muscles in the shoulders and upper back, this pose strengthens the wrists and improves the range of movement in the shoulder joints. It can also be beneficial for those who spend a great deal of time at a computer.

1   **BEGINNER**

1 Begin in a comfortable standing position.

2 Relax your shoulders and allow your hands to hang down by your sides.

3 Reach your fists behind your back so that they touch, rotating your shoulders inward.

4 Inhale, draw the crown of your head up and lengthen your spine; exhale and press your knuckles together.

Keep your shoulders relaxed

Press your shoulder blades together

Press your knuckles together

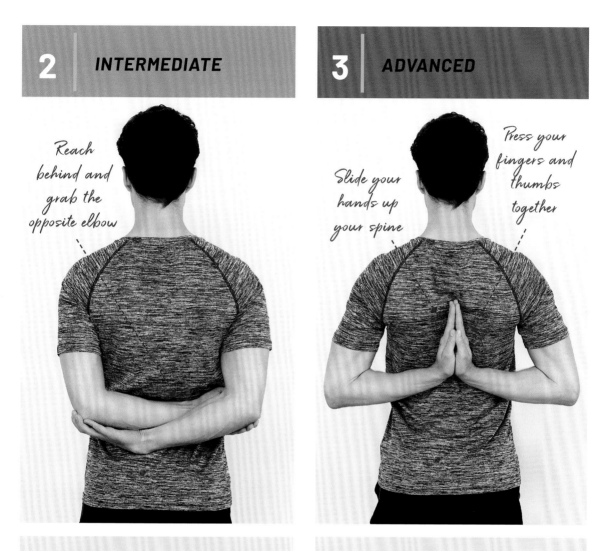

Reach behind and grab the opposite elbow

Slide your hands up your spine

Press your fingers and thumbs together

INTERMEDIATE

1 Begin as before.
2 Reach behind your back and grab the opposite elbow.
3 Inhale, draw the crown of your head up, and lengthen your spine; exhale and pull your elbows closer together.
4 Repeat, this time interlacing the arms the other way around.

ADVANCED

1 Begin as before.
2 Reach behind your back to press your fingers together.
3 Slide your hands up your spine while pressing into your hands and fingers.
4 Inhale, draw the crown of your head up, and lengthen your spine; exhale and press your hands closer together.

COW FACE ARMS POSE

Cow face arms pose focuses on flexibility in the shoulders, armpits, triceps, and chest. Opening the chest can help improve breathing, circulation, and metabolism as well as reducing stress and anxiety.

1 Begin in a comfortable position, either seated or standing.

2 Reach your left arm up over your head and bend it at the elbow; catch your tricep with your right hand and gently pull it down.

3 Inhale and lengthen your spine; exhale and press down into your tricep to intensify the stretch. Repeat on the other side.

Gently pull down your tricep with your other hand

Bend your arm at the elbow, reaching down behind your head

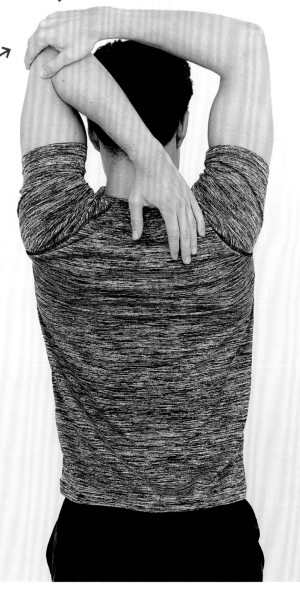

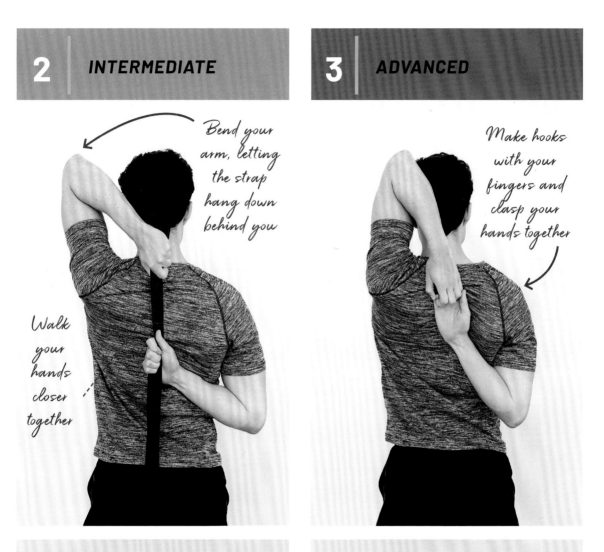

Bend your arm, letting the strap hang down behind you

Walk your hands closer together

Make hooks with your fingers and clasp your hands together

1 Begin as before.

2 With a strap in your left hand, bend your arm, letting the strap hang down behind your back.

3 Bend your right arm and grab the strap. It doesn't matter how far apart your hands are.

4 Inhale to lengthen your spine and exhale to walk your hands closer together.

5 Release the strap. Repeat on the other side.

1 Begin as before.

2 Once you are able to bring your hands behind your back comfortably using the strap, practice without the strap.

3 Make hooks with your fingers and clasp your hands together.

4 Inhale to lengthen your spine and exhale to clasp your hands closer together. Repeat on the other side.

REVERSE PLANK

The stages of this pose progress from reverse table top to reverse plank with one leg raised. It stretches the shoulders and all along the front of the body. It also strengthens the arms, wrists, and legs, as well as engaging the abdominal muscles.

1 Begin by sitting with your legs straight out in front.

2 Bend your knees so that your feet are flat on the floor. Leave about 1ft between your hips and your feet.

3 Frame your hips about 1ft behind, with your fingertips facing your feet.

4 Inhale and lift your hips while at the same time pressing down firmly onto your hands and feet.

5 Move your shoulder blades closer to one another to open your chest.

6 Inhale to prepare; exhale to push your hips up farther and open your shoulders more.

7 Ensure your neck stays neutral, or if it is more comfortable, gently let the head tip back.

8 To come out of the pose, drop your hips back down to the floor.

Keep your thighs and upper body parallel to the floor

Make sure your knees are at 90 degrees

Keep your wrists under your shoulders

Point your fingertips toward your feet

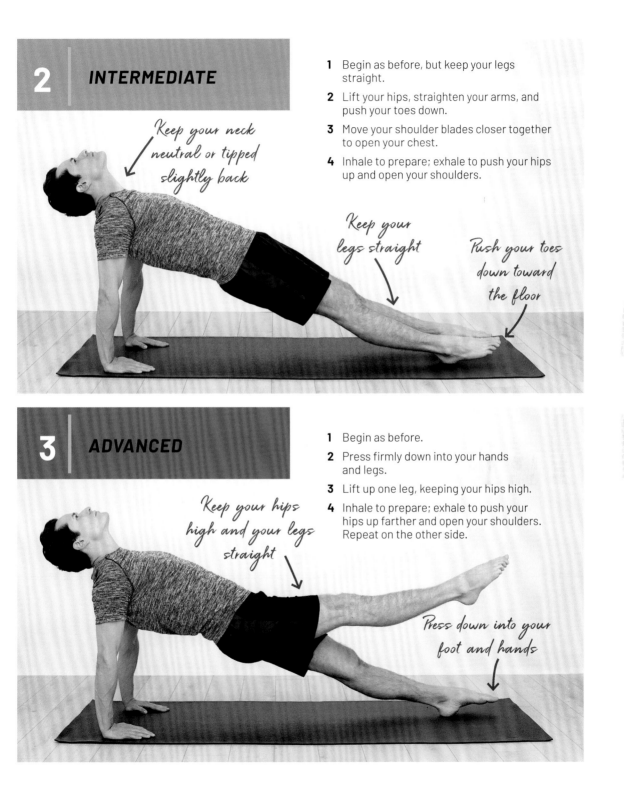

2 | INTERMEDIATE

Keep your neck neutral or tipped slightly back

1 Begin as before, but keep your legs straight.
2 Lift your hips, straighten your arms, and push your toes down.
3 Move your shoulder blades closer together to open your chest.
4 Inhale to prepare; exhale to push your hips up and open your shoulders.

Keep your legs straight

Push your toes down toward the floor

3 | ADVANCED

Keep your hips high and your legs straight

1 Begin as before.
2 Press firmly down into your hands and legs.
3 Lift up one leg, keeping your hips high.
4 Inhale to prepare; exhale to push your hips up farther and open your shoulders. Repeat on the other side.

Press down into your foot and hands

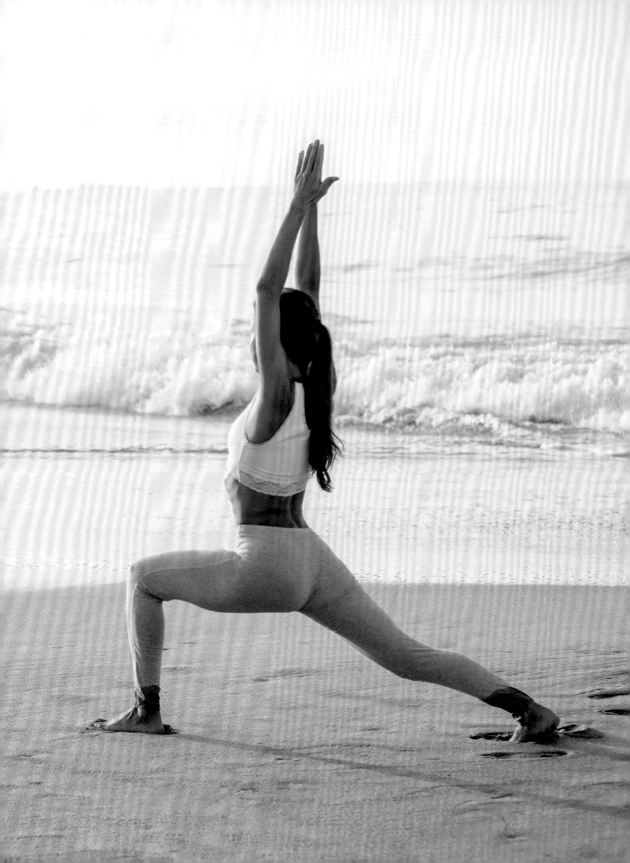

4

HIP AND LEG FLEXORS

A sedentary lifestyle and, conversely, running can cause tightness in the legs and hips, and restricted hip mobility can lead to lower back pain and knee problems. The root chakra is located at the base of the spine and is where we ground ourselves into the earth and anchor our energy into the world. Its key characteristics are security, safety, survival, support, and the foundation for living our lives. Therefore, working the hips can promote both physical and emotional flexibility. In this section we will work on stretching the quadriceps, hip flexors, hamstrings, and glutes. Opening up the hips and legs is also important for backbends, so we will focus on this section first.

HERO'S POSE

Hero's pose is a classic, seated yoga pose that stretches the thighs and ankles while improving posture. It is beneficial for the mobility and health of knees, ankles, and thighs and provides internal thigh rotation. As it's such a deep stretch for the knees, take the pose slowly and use props as needed to get safely in and out of the pose.

1 | **BEGINNER**

1 Begin by kneeling on the floor with a block on its lowest setting just underneath your sit bones.

2 With the tops of your feet on the floor, sit upright with your hands on your thighs.

3 Inhale to lengthen your spine; exhale to sink deeper into your hips and down into the floor.

4 To come out of the pose, lean forward and prop yourself up with your hands as you slide onto all fours.

5 If you feel any pinching or pain, back out of the pose as above and place the blocks at a higher level and try again.

Sit upright with your hands on the front of your thighs

Place the tops of your feet on the floor on either side of the block

Place the block just under the sit bones

1 Begin by kneeling on the floor (use a folded blanket if you need more padding).

2 Open your feet slightly wider than your hips, keeping the tops of your feet flat on the floor and your big toes facing toward one another.

3 Lean your torso forward as you reach your hands back to draw your calves outward to make room for your thighs and hips.

4 Sit between your feet with your heels and shins alongside your hips and upper thighs, your feet directly in line with your shins, and let your hands rest on your thighs.

5 Drop your shoulders away from your ears and lengthen your tailbone to the floor.

6 Inhale to lengthen your spine; exhale to sink deeper into your hips and down into the floor.

7 Come out of the pose as before.

Sit up straight and draw your shoulder blades down your spine

Stretch out your chest

Keep the tops of your feet flat on the floor with your big toes facing one another

Keep your feet directly in line with your shins

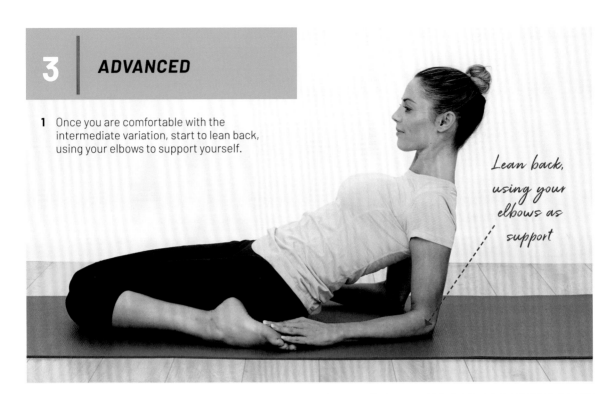

3 | ADVANCED

1 Once you are comfortable with the intermediate variation, start to lean back, using your elbows to support yourself.

Lean back, using your elbows as support

2 Start to lean back farther, until you are resting your upper back and head on the floor. You can move your hands up and over your head, grabbing onto the opposite elbow.

3 Inhale to lengthen your spine; exhale to sink deeper into the floor.

4 To come out of the pose, prop yourself up on your elbows and use your core and hands to lift your upper body.

Rest your upper back and head on the floor

Place your arms above your head, grabbing the opposite elbow

CRESCENT LUNGE

This dynamic standing yoga pose stretches the hip flexors, quads, calves, and ankles while strengthening the legs and improving stability. It also stretches the chest, shoulders, and back, increases energy, and reduces fatigue.

1 Begin in table-top position (*see page 27*).

2 Step your right foot forward between your hands with your back knee on the floor.

3 Bend your front leg to 90 degrees, stacking your knee over your ankle and your foot facing forward.

4 Square your hips so that they face forward, and squeeze your back glute. Place your hands on your hips.

5 Inhale to lengthen your spine; exhale to sink deeper into the lunge.

6 Draw your front ribs in and engage your core.

7 To come out of the pose, plant your hands down on the floor and step your front foot back to table-top position. Repeat on the other side.

Keep your gaze neutral and look straight ahead

Stack your knee over the heel of your front foot

Square your hips so they face forward

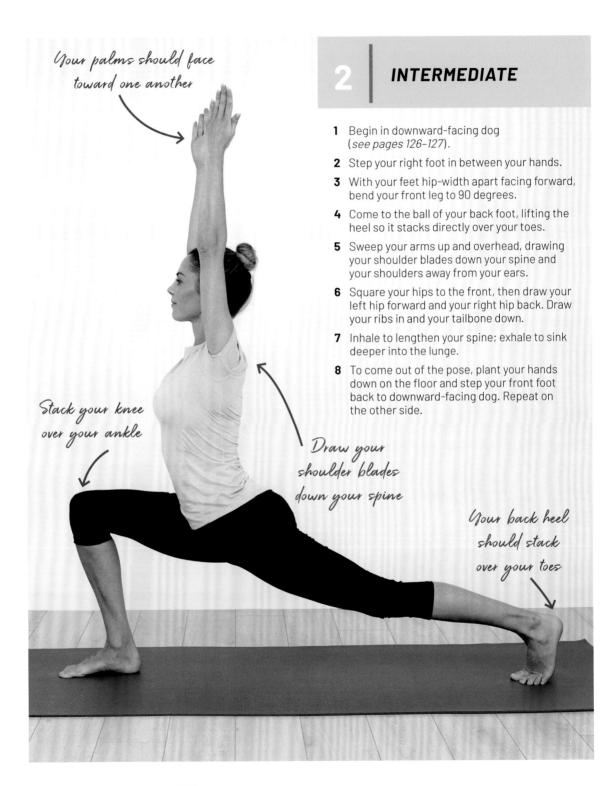

Your palms should face toward one another

1   Begin in downward-facing dog
    (*see pages 126–127*).

2   Step your right foot in between your hands.

3   With your feet hip-width apart facing forward,
    bend your front leg to 90 degrees.

4   Come to the ball of your back foot, lifting the
    heel so it stacks directly over your toes.

5   Sweep your arms up and overhead, drawing
    your shoulder blades down your spine and
    your shoulders away from your ears.

6   Square your hips to the front, then draw your
    left hip forward and your right hip back. Draw
    your ribs in and your tailbone down.

7   Inhale to lengthen your spine; exhale to sink
    deeper into the lunge.

8   To come out of the pose, plant your hands
    down on the floor and step your front foot
    back to downward-facing dog. Repeat on
    the other side.

Stack your knee over your ankle

Draw your shoulder blades down your spine

Your back heel should stack over your toes

1. Begin as before.
2. In crescent lunge with your arms above your head, start to bend back, tilting your head to look toward the back of the room.
3. Engage your core, draw your tailbone down and your ribs in to protect your spine in the backbend.
4. Inhale to lengthen your spine and reach your arms up; exhale to reach back and extend your spine back farther.
5. To come out of the pose, plant your hands down on the floor and step your front foot back to downward-facing dog, sending your hips up toward the sky.

3 | ADVANCED

Bend backward and tilt your head toward the back of the room

Engage your core and your legs

Draw your tailbone down and your ribs in

| NEXT LEVEL | To get a deeper stretch for your toes and foot, shift your back heel forward so your heel is over your toes. |

BOUND ANGLE POSE

The bound angle pose or cobbler's pose is one of the best external hip openers. It stimulates the internal organs, stretches the inner thighs, groin, and knees, and soothes menstrual discomfort and sciatica.

1 Begin by sitting with your legs straight out in front, keeping your spine long.

2 Bend both knees and press the soles of your feet together.

3 Take two blocks and place them underneath your knees for more support (at a low or high setting).

4 Draw your heels in toward your groin.

5 With your hands on your feet as if you were holding an open book, rotate your feet outward.

6 Sit up straight and extend the full length of your spine to the crown of your head.

7 Inhale to lengthen your spine; exhale to pull your knees down toward the floor.

8 To release, draw your knees up to the sky and extend your legs out in front.

Sit up straight and extend the full length of your spine

Draw your heels toward your groin

Press the soles of your feet together

2 | INTERMEDIATE

1 Repeat as before, this time without using blocks.

2 Inhale to lengthen your spine; exhale to pull your knees down toward the floor.

3 Release as before.

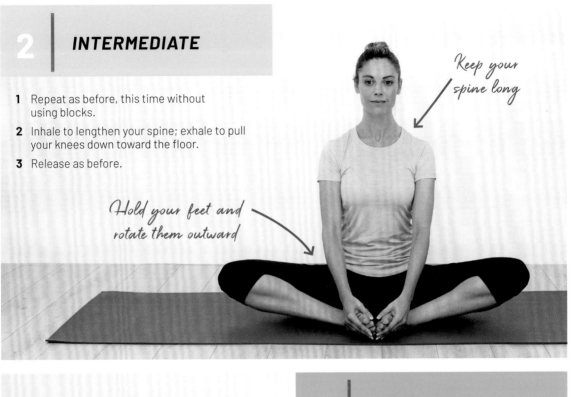

Keep your spine long

Hold your feet and rotate them outward

1 Start to bend at the hips into a forward fold without rounding your spine or shoulders.

2 Move your chest toward your toes, keeping your torso and spine long.

3 Inhale to lengthen your spine; exhale to fold deeper toward the floor.

4 To release, inhale to lift your chest up and draw your knees up toward the sky.

3 | ADVANCED

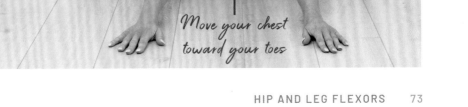

Don't round your spine or shoulders

Move your chest toward your toes

SEATED WIDE-LEGGED STRADDLE POSE

This pose stretches the inner thighs and hamstrings and can help to ease sciatica and arthritis. It also strengthens the back and spine, stimulates the abdominal organs, works the core muscles and relaxes the brain.

1 | BEGINNER

1 Begin by sitting with your legs straight out in front.

2 Open your legs to about 90 degrees, with your hands behind your back for support or in front of the hips, and your feet flexed with your toes pointing up to the sky (and your thighs rotated outward).

3 Draw your kneecaps up toward your hips to protect your knees.

4 Keep your torso long and extended.

5 Inhale and exhale deeply to keep your spine long and neutral.

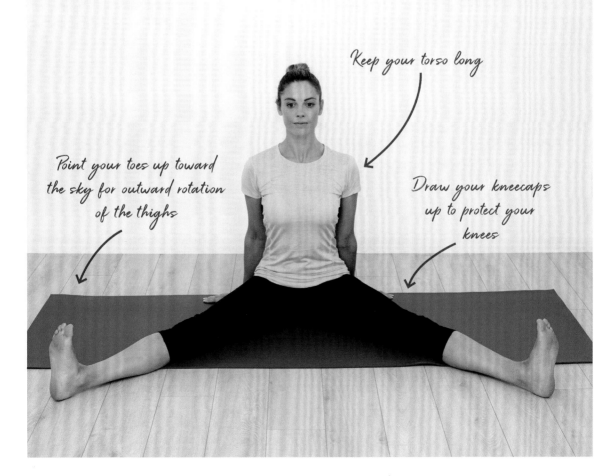

Keep your torso long

Point your toes up toward the sky for outward rotation of the thighs

Draw your kneecaps up to protect your knees

2 | INTERMEDIATE

1 Begin as before and then start to bend at the hips into a forward fold, walking your hands forward.

2 Keep your toes pointing up toward the sky for outward rotation of the thighs.

3 Focus on moving from the hip joints and maintaining the length of your torso; you can prop yourself up on your forearms if you need to.

4 Inhale to lengthen your spine; exhale to fold toward the floor, keeping your spine long and straight.

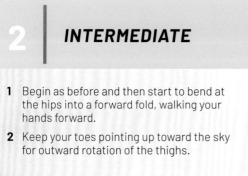

Bring your belly to the floor first

3 | ADVANCED

1 Begin as before.

2 Once your belly touches the floor, bend your knees slightly, slide your arms under your thighs, fold to the floor, and straighten your legs again.

3 Inhale to lengthen your spine; exhale to fold toward the floor, keeping your spine long and straight.

When your belly touches the floor, slide your arms under your thighs and fold forward

FIGURE FOUR POSE

The figure four pose strengthens the quads, ankles, and foot muscles. It also stretches the outer hip and glute muscles and relieves lower back tension. The standing posture tones the core and allows you to practice balance and mental concentration.

1 Lie on your back and bring your knees toward your chest.

2 Cross your left ankle over your right knee.

3 Loop your hands behind your right thigh and gently pull your legs closer to your chest so you can feel a stretch in your outer right hip.

4 Flex your feet, especially your left foot, to protect your knees.

5 Inhale to prepare; exhale to pull your knees into your chest. Repeat on the other side.

Flex your feet to protect your knees

Pull your legs closer to your chest to increase the stretch

1 In a seated position, bend your knees into your chest, keeping your feet on the floor.

2 Cross your left ankle over your right thigh close to the knee.

3 Support your upper body with your hands behind your hips.

4 Flex your right foot to protect your knee.

5 Inhale to prepare; exhale to fold deeper, bringing your chest closer to your ankle. Repeat on the other side.

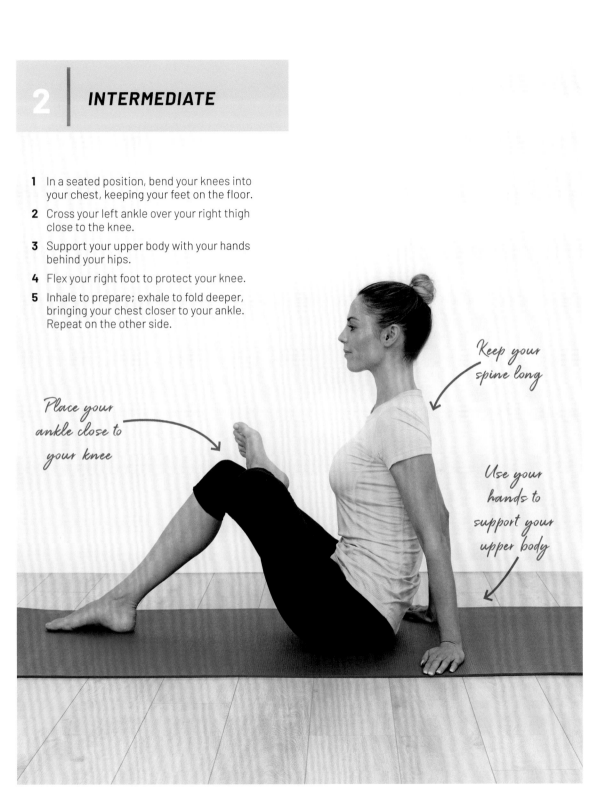

Place your ankle close to your knee

Keep your spine long

Use your hands to support your upper body

3 | ADVANCED A

1 In a standing position bend your knees slightly.

2 Taking a moment to focus, shift your weight to your right leg and lift up your left foot.

3 Cross your left ankle over your right thigh just above the knee, keeping your right knee bent.

4 Bring your hands to your heart.

5 Inhale to lengthen your spine; exhale to sink your hips down a little deeper while opening the top knee down to the floor. Repeat on the other side.

Flex the foot of the leg you have lifted

Cross your leg over the opposite thigh just above the knee

Keep the knee of your supporting leg bent

4 ADVANCED B

1 Begin as before.

2 To go deeper into the pose, start to fold forward over your thigh, placing your hands on the floor.

3 Inhale to lengthen your spine; exhale to fold down a little deeper, bringing your chest closer to your ankle and shin. Repeat on the other side.

Fold forward over your thigh

Cross your ankle over your thigh just above the knee

Place your hands on the floor

NEXT LEVEL

Try bending the bottom leg more to bring the top leg closer to the chest to intensify the stretch.

LIZARD LUNGE

The lizard lunge is great for opening the hips, hip flexors, quads, and hamstrings. It can be an active or passive stretch depending on what you need. It strengthens and tones the legs while releasing the hips and improving the flexibility of the ligaments.

1   Begin in table-top position (*see page 27*), with your hands resting on blocks at a low or high setting, whichever is the most suitable for you. Stack your shoulders over your wrists and your hips over your knees.

2   Step your right foot up to the outside of your right hand.

3   Slide your left knee back a little and slowly sink your weight down into your hips.

4   Inhale to lengthen your spine; exhale to sink deeper into your hips, keeping them square.

5   To come out of the pose, press your weight into your hands and step your right leg back to meet your left. Repeat on the other side.

Keep your hips square

Place your foot on the outside of your hand

Roll over the top of the knee so you're not pressing directly on the joint

2 | INTERMEDIATE

1 Begin as before.

2 Tuck your toes under and lift your left knee off the floor, straightening your leg.

3 Inhale to lengthen your spine; exhale to sink into your hips. Repeat on the other side.

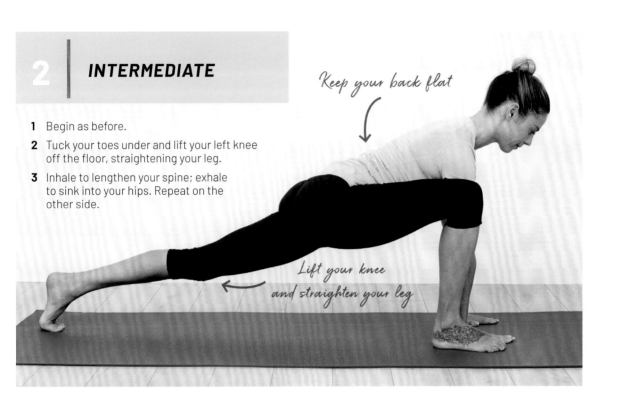

Keep your back flat

Lift your knee and straighten your leg

3 | ADVANCED

1 Begin as before.

2 If you want to go deeper, lower one forearm at a time to the floor.

3 Inhale to lengthen your spine; exhale to sink deeper into your hips, keeping them square. Repeat on the other side.

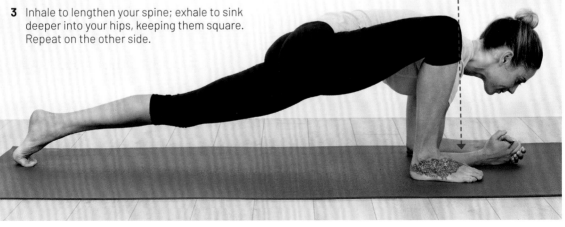

Lower your forearms to the floor, one at a time

HALF PIGEON POSE

The half pigeon pose is one of the final poses in a yoga practice. Used to open hips, hip flexors, and quads, it can provide relief from sciatica and back pain. It calms the mind and allows you to turn your thoughts inward for reflection.

1   From downward-facing dog (*see pages 126–127*), bring your right foot toward your left hand, and your right knee toward your right hand.

2   Flex your right foot and make sure that your shin is parallel to the front of your mat.

3   Set your hips to a block, with most of your right hip resting on the block and your left leg straight out behind you.

4   This should be an intense hip stretch; don't force your legs down into the pose—take it slowly and breathe through it.

5   Look back to see if your rear leg is in a straight line from your middle.

6   Inhale to lengthen your spine; exhale to sink into your hips, keeping them square.

7   To come out of the pose, plant your hands down by your sides and come back into downward-facing dog. Repeat on the other side.

Use your hands to frame your hips and keep your torso upright

Rest most of your hip on the block with the other leg straight out behind you

Make sure your shin is parallel to the front of the mat

INTERMEDIATE

1 Begin as before, this time without a block under the hips.

2 Square your hips then pull your left hip forward and your right hip back.

3 Inhale to lengthen your spine; exhale to sink deeper into your hips, keeping them square to the front. Repeat on the other side.

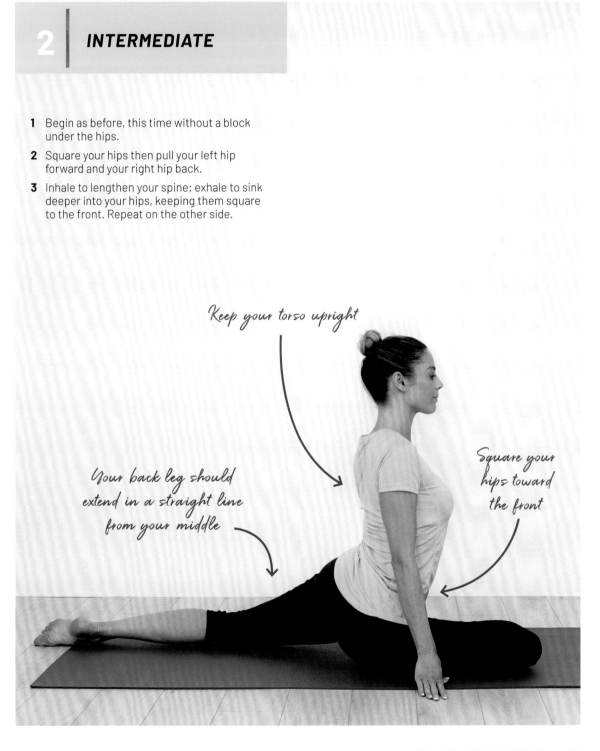

Keep your torso upright

Your back leg should extend in a straight line from your middle

Square your hips toward the front

3 | ADVANCED

1 Begin as before.
2 Start to walk your hands to the front of the mat and fold forward, resting your torso over your right leg.

Rest your torso over your front leg

Support yourself with your forearms

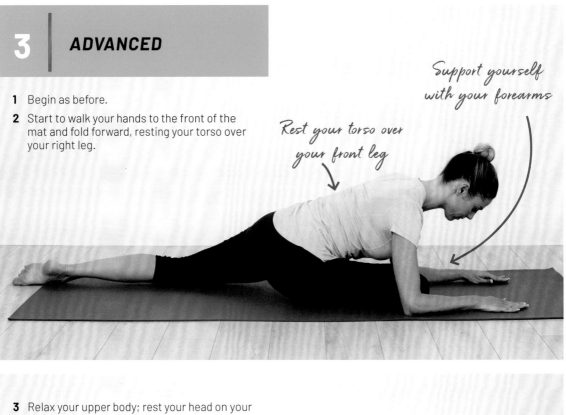

3 Relax your upper body; rest your head on your forearms, or your forehead on the floor with your arms extended straight out in front.

4 Inhale to lengthen your spine; exhale to sink deeper into your hips, keeping them square to the front. Repeat on the other side.

Relax your upper body

Extend your arms out in front

LOTUS POSE

Traditionally practiced to calm the mind and prepare you for meditation, the lotus pose stretches the knees, ankles, and hips and improves flexibility. It also strengthens the spine and upper back and promotes good posture by keeping the back straight.

BEGINNER

1   Sit on the floor with your legs extended straight out in front.

2   Bend your left knee and draw your left heel to your right glute underneath your right leg.

3   Bend your right knee and hug it into your chest.

4   Bring your right ankle to the crease of your left hip so the sole of your right foot is facing upward.

5   Relax your hands onto your knees, either with your palms facing down (for introspection/grounding), or facing up (for receiving).

6   Relax your shoulders and draw your shoulder blades down your spine, sitting up tall.

7   Hold for as long as you wish for your meditation or breathing practice.

8   To come out of the pose, uncross your right ankle. Repeat on the other side.

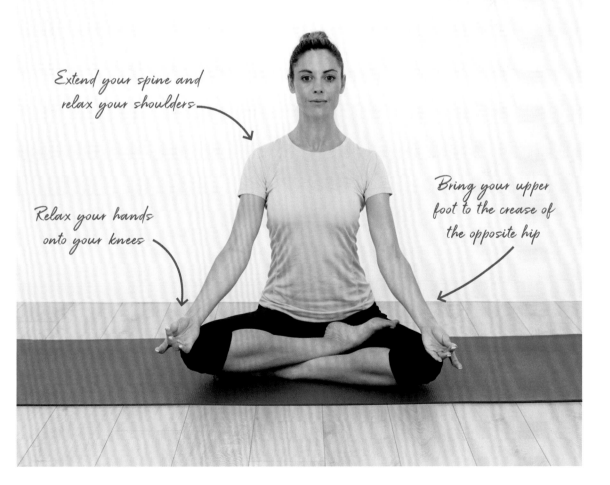

Extend your spine and relax your shoulders

Relax your hands onto your knees

Bring your upper foot to the crease of the opposite hip

1 Begin as before.

2 Bend your right knee to your chest and then bring your right foot to the crease of your left hip with the sole of your foot facing upward.

3 Bend your left knee and cross your left ankle over the top of your right shin in full lotus position. The sole of your left foot should face upward, with the top of the foot and the ankle resting on your hip crease.

4 With your hands on your knees in your preferred position, relax your shoulders and draw your shoulder blades down your spine, sitting up tall.

5 Repeat with your legs crossed the opposite way.

Remember to relax your shoulders and sit up tall

To protect your joints, do not force your ankles to cross over

3 | ADVANCED

1 Begin as before.

2 Once in full lotus, reach behind your back with both arms. If you wish, you can hook your index and middle fingers around your toes (right hand to right toes and left hand to left toes).

3 Hold for as long as you wish for your meditation or breathing practice.

Reach around behind your back with both arms

Remember to alternate the leg crosses when you practice this pose

SPLITS POSE

The front splits with the legs stretching out in opposite directions symbolizes the great distance traveled by the god Hanuman. In Hindu mythology, Hanuman took a mighty leap all the way from the south of India to the Himalayas to save his king's brother—thus the pose represents devotion and strength. The pose is physically challenging, and the three variations—half splits, full splits with blocks, and full splits/standing splits—offer a gradual progression.

1 | BEGINNER

1 Begin in table-top position (*see page 27*).

2 Step your right foot forward in between your hands.

3 Straighten your right leg and flex your foot; engage your quads to protect your knees.

4 Keep your hips square and stacked over your back knee.

5 Inhale to lengthen your spine and exhale to fold down over your front thigh.

6 To come out of the pose, step your right leg back and come back to table-top position. Repeat on the other side.

When you exhale, fold down over your front thigh

Keep your hips square and stacked over your back knee

Straighten your leg and flex your foot

2 | INTERMEDIATE

1 Begin as before, and come into half splits.
2 Hold onto blocks either side of your hips at a low or high setting.
3 Start to slide your right heel forward as you bring your hips closer to the floor.
4 Square your hips to the front, and squeeze your left glute. Flex your right foot.

5 Inhale to lengthen your spine and exhale to press down farther.
6 To come out of the pose, press down into the blocks with your hands to lift your hips up. Repeat on the other side.

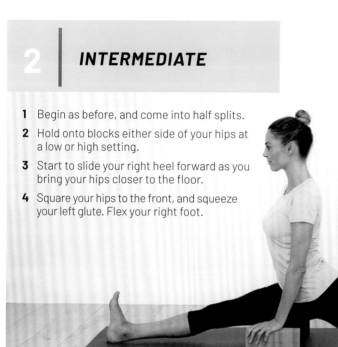

Press down on the blocks with your hands to take the weight off your legs

1 Begin as before, and come into half splits, this time without blocks.
2 Lower your hips down to the floor with your hands supporting you on either side.
3 Slowly begin to extend your front leg.
4 Inhale to lengthen your spine and exhale to press down farther.

3 | ADVANCED

5 To come out of the pose, press down into the floor with your hands to lift your hips.

If your legs/ hips don't reach the floor, place your hands by your sides

Protect your knees by engaging your quads

MIDDLE SPLITS

The middle splits is another challenging pose and it takes a great deal of practice to develop the flexibility needed to achieve it. It provides a deep stretch for the thighs, opens the hip flexors, and develops perseverance as you take your time to progress through the three stages.

1 | *BEGINNER*

1 Begin in table-top position (*see page 27*), walk your knees out to the side, and flex your feet outward.

2 Come down onto your forearms and start to slide your legs away from one another.

3 Inhale to lengthen your spine; exhale to slide your knees farther away from one another and engage your hips.

4 To come out of the pose, slide your forearms forward, bring your legs together behind you, and come into child's pose (*see page 54*).

Maintain a neutral spine

The soles of your feet should be at 90 degrees to your shins

Keep your shins parallel

2 | INTERMEDIATE

1 Begin in a seated wide-legged straddle pose (*see pages 74–75*).

2 Bend your left knee into your groin. Keeping your right leg straight, flex your right foot so that your toes are pointing upward.

3 Stretch your right leg out to increase the stretch in your left hip flexor.

4 Inhale to lengthen your spine; exhale to fold your belly toward the floor.

5 To come out of the pose, inhale to bring your spine upright and straighten your left leg to come back into wide-legged straddle pose. Repeat on the other side.

Point your toes upward

You can place your hands on the floor for stability

1 Begin in a standing wide-legged forward fold (*see pages 44–45*).

2 Putting pressure into your hands, slide your feet away from one another, gradually bringing your thighs down to the floor.

3 Come onto your forearms.

4 Inhale to prepare; exhale to bring your hips closer to the floor.

5 To come out of the pose, shift your torso forward and bring your legs together behind you until you are lying on the floor on your belly.

3 | ADVANCED

Don't force your legs down to the floor

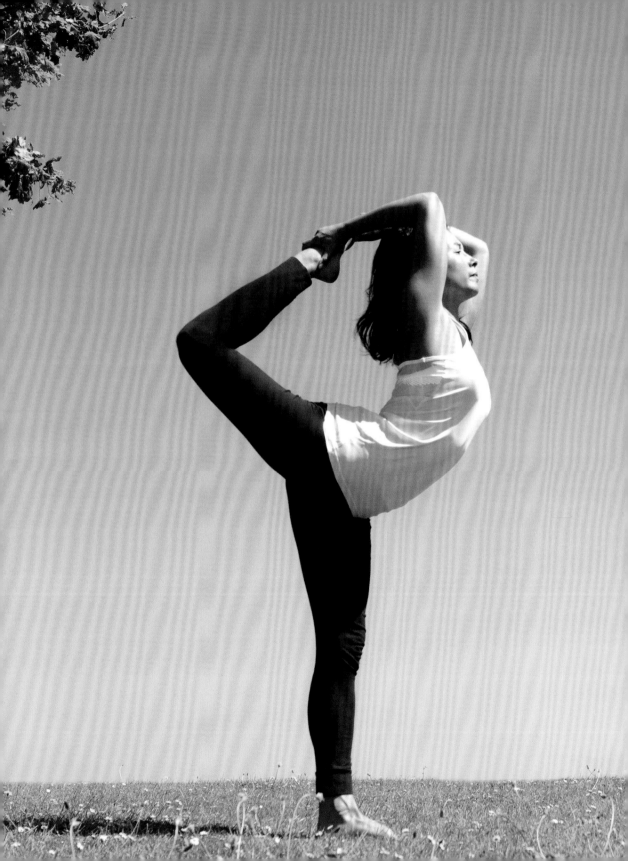

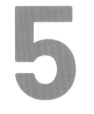

BACKBENDS

In our daily lives we spend so much time sitting down and bending forward that our spines begin to lose their natural flexion. Practicing backbends regularly will reverse this process and also strengthen and increase flexibility all down the back of the body, including the legs, glutes, and the muscles surrounding the ribs and torso. These postures compress the kidneys, and when released, the flow of new blood flushes toxins from the body. Backbends are known for their ability to relieve stress and anxiety as well as improving posture. Opening the front of the body stretches the abs and opens the lungs, helping to improve breathing and reduce fatigue. Other benefits of backbends include the relief of back and neck pain, improved sleep patterns, and an increase in confidence as you progress through the stages of each posture.

COBRA POSE

The cobra pose opens the heart and chest while strengthening the back muscles. It prepares your body for deeper backbends and can help to reverse the effects of hours spent hunched in front of a computer. It also tones the glutes and strengthens the arms.

1 Lie on your stomach on the floor.

2 Place your palms on the floor next to your ribs with your fingertips in line with the front of your shoulders.

3 Hug your elbows to your sides.

4 Press your palms firmly into the floor and begin to lift your chest.

5 Maintain a long, neutral neck; try not to force your head back.

6 Keep your shoulders away from your ears.

7 Extend your legs back and keep them engaged.

8 Engage your back muscles to lift your chest off the floor; put little weight in the fingertips.

9 Inhale to lengthen your spine; exhale to lift your chest farther off the floor.

10 To release, lower yourself to the floor, keeping your torso long.

Maintain a long, neutral neck and keep your shoulders down

Keep your legs engaged

Make sure your fingertips are in line with the front of your shoulders

2 | INTERMEDIATE

1 Begin as before.
2 Press your palms into the floor and lift up your chest; slowly straighten your arms.
3 Keep your legs engaged, and your shoulders away from your ears.
4 Inhale to lengthen your spine; exhale to press into your hands and open your chest farther.
5 Release as before.

Use your back muscles to stop yourself pushing down into your hands and shoulders

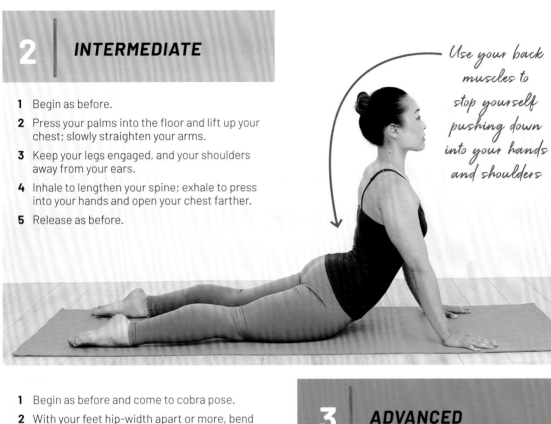

1 Begin as before and come to cobra pose.
2 With your feet hip-width apart or more, bend one knee at a time toward your head.
3 Bend both knees at the same time and press down into your hands, reaching for your head.
4 Inhale to lengthen your spine; exhale to press into your hands.
5 To release, straighten your legs and lower yourself slowly to the floor.

3 | ADVANCED

Tilt your head back slowly and engage your core

Start by bending one knee at a time

LOCUST POSE

The locust pose increases flexibility all along the back of the body, including the spine, legs, glutes, and the muscles surrounding the ribs and torso, and also helps to repair the spinal cord. It opens the lungs, improves breathing, and can relieve stress and fatigue caused by slouching forward.

1 | **BEGINNER**

1 Start by lying on your stomach; place a towel under your face and/or your pelvis if you wish.

2 With your arms by your sides, and your palms facing down next to your hips, take a couple of breaths in and out.

3 When you are ready, exhale, press down into your hands, and lift your head and torso, engaging your back muscles.

4 Engage your glutes and legs so they stay in contact with the floor.

5 Draw your shoulders away from your ears and your shoulder blades down your spine.

6 Hold for a couple of breaths; on the last exhale, slowly lower your chest down to the floor.

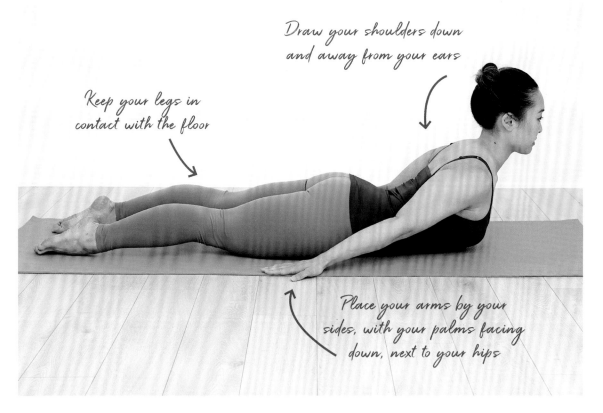

Draw your shoulders down and away from your ears

Keep your legs in contact with the floor

Place your arms by your sides, with your palms facing down, next to your hips

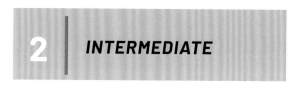

1 Begin as before.

2 This time, lift your arms up by your sides at the same time as lifting your legs.

3 Hold for a couple of breaths; on the last exhale, slowly lower your chest and legs down to the floor.

Engage your back muscles, glutes, and legs

Lower your back down to the floor on the exhale

Lift your arms and your legs at the same time

3 | ADVANCED

1 Begin as before.

2 Move your arms and elbows under your torso with your hands touching the floor, palms facing downward; you may have to round your spine a little to do this. Take a couple of breaths in and out through your nose.

3 Inhale to lengthen your spine and prepare; exhale to press down into your hands and lift up your legs as high as possible, engaging your back muscles. You can start by lifting one leg up at a time.

4 Hold at the top for a couple of breaths; on your next exhale, slowly lower your legs down to the floor.

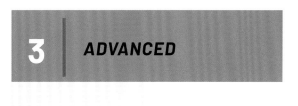

Lift your legs as high as possible, engaging your back muscles

Move your elbows and arms under your torso

Place your hands on the floor with your palms facing downward

NEXT LEVEL

Press your hands firmly into the ground and lift your legs higher off the ground so they are perpendicular to the floor.

BOW POSE

The bow pose stretches all along the front of the body, from the ankles, thighs, hips, hip flexors, core, chest, and throat, while strengthening the back muscles. It opens the shoulders, improves posture, and stimulates the abdominal organs and neck.

1 For the half bow pose, start by lying on your stomach; place a towel under your pelvis to provide more padding if you wish.

2 Come onto your forearms to lift up your chest.

3 Bend your left leg and reach back with your right hand to grab onto the inside of your left foot/ankle.

4 Press into your left forearm to lift your chest.

5 Holding onto your left ankle, press your foot into your hand to lift your chest.

6 Inhale to lengthen your spine; exhale to kick back into your leg to open your shoulders farther and lift your chest higher.

7 To come out of the pose, relax your leg and let go of your left foot/ankle.

8 Repeat on the other side.

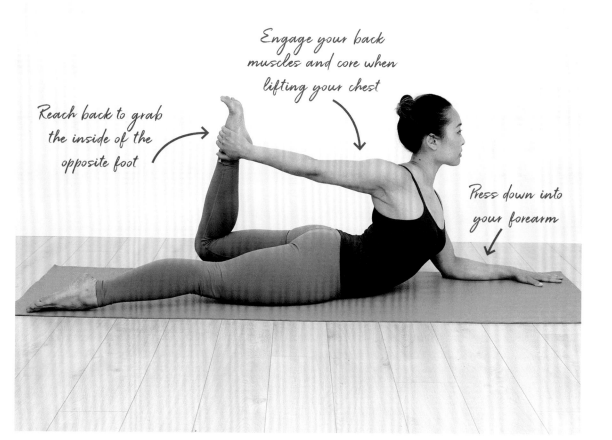

Engage your back muscles and core when lifting your chest

Reach back to grab the inside of the opposite foot

Press down into your forearm

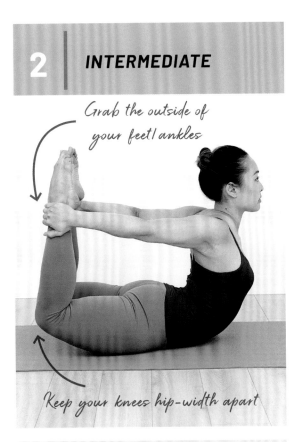

Grab the outside of your feet/ankles

Keep your knees hip-width apart

1. Begin as before, with your hands by your hips and your palms facing up.

2. Exhale, bend your knees, and bring your heels as close as possible to your glutes.

3. Reach back with your hands to grab your feet.

4. Lift your heels away from your glutes and your thighs away from the floor. This will pull your head and chest off the floor.

5. Engage your core and back muscles and draw your shoulders away from your ears.

6. Inhale to lengthen your spine; exhale to kick back into your legs to open your shoulders farther and lift your chest higher.

7. To come out of the pose, relax your legs, let go of your feet/ankles, and lower your chest.

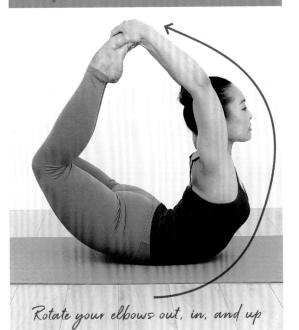

Rotate your elbows out, in, and up

1. Begin as before.

2. Bend your knees and bring your heels to your glutes.

3. Flex your feet out to the side and grab hold of the top of each foot.

4. Hold the tops of the feet until your arms are up and overhead.

5. Press your feet into your hands to lift your chest.

6. Inhale to lengthen your spine; exhale to kick back into your feet to open your shoulders farther and lift your chest higher.

7. To come out of the pose, relax your legs, let go of your feet/ankles, and slowly lower your chest to the floor.

CAMEL POSE

The camel pose increases spine flexibility, stimulates the nervous system, improves circulation, and stimulates the thyroid. It can also help to reduce blood pressure and provides relief from stress and anxiety by decreasing tension in your neck, back, and shoulders.

1 | **BEGINNER**

1. Kneel with your legs hip-width apart and your thighs perpendicular to the floor.

2. Rotate your thighs inward, press your shins into the floor, and tuck in your toes to elevate your ankles.

3. Place two blocks on the outside of your feet, directly in line with your ankles, at a low or high setting.

4. Draw your shoulders down and away from your ears.

5. Push down into the blocks to lift your chest higher; stay in the pose for 5–10 breaths.

6. To come out of the pose, place your hands on your lower back, engage your core, and bring your head and torso back to neutral.

7. Rest in child's pose (*see page 54*).

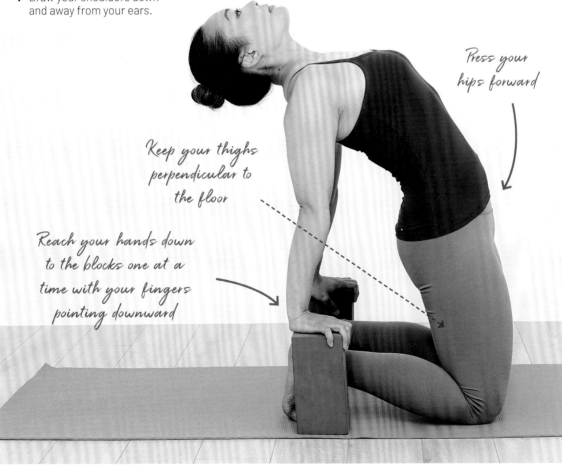

Press your hips forward

Keep your thighs perpendicular to the floor

Reach your hands down to the blocks one at a time with your fingers pointing downward

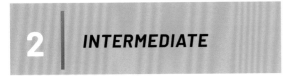

1 Begin as before, this time without blocks.

2 Bring your hands to the back of your hips with your fingers pointing down.

3 Draw your shoulders down and away from your ears.

4 Lift your chest up, lean back slightly, and reach one hand at a time down to your ankles.

5 Press your hips forward and lift your chest up. Stay in the pose for 5–10 breaths.

6 To come out of the pose, place your hands on your lower back, engage your core, and bring your head and torso back to neutral.

7 Rest in child's pose (*see page 54*) for a couple of breaths to center.

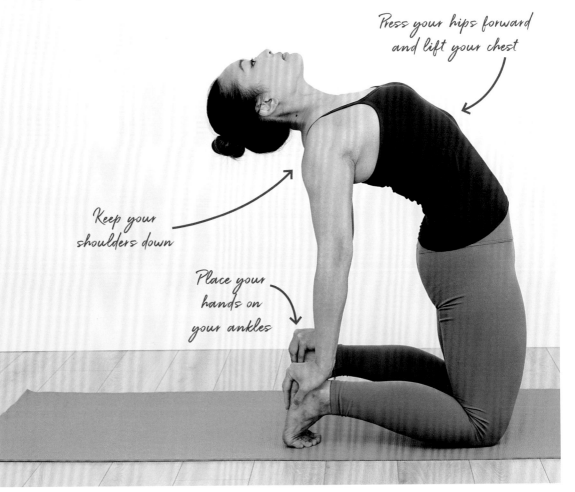

Press your hips forward and lift your chest

Keep your shoulders down

Place your hands on your ankles

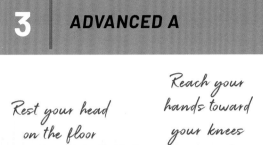

3 | ADVANCED A

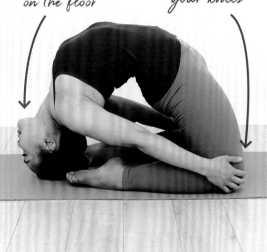

Rest your head on the floor

Reach your hands toward your knees

1. Begin as before.
2. Untuck your toes so the tops of your feet are on the floor. Start with your hands on your lower back. Inhale to lengthen your spine; exhale to arch your spine back. Press your hips forward and walk your hands down your thighs as you extend your spine down until your head comes into contact with the floor.
3. Extend your hands toward your knees and stay in the pose for a couple of breaths in and out through your nose.
4. To come out of the pose, engage your back muscles and glutes and on the exhale, start to lift your head off the ground and walk your hands back up to your lower back.
5. Sit back on your heels and rest your hands on your thighs to center.

4 | ADVANCED B

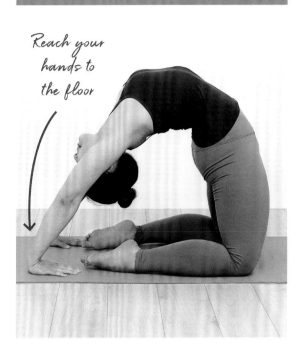

Reach your hands to the floor

1. Begin as before.
2. Untuck your toes so the tops of your feet are on the floor. Inhale, lift your arms up and overhead, and on the exhale, start to reach back and arch your spine from your shoulders and upper back. Press your hips forward and lean back until your hands touch the floor.
3. Inhale to lengthen your spine; exhale to go a little deeper into the backbend.
4. To come out of the pose, engage your back muscles and glutes and on the exhale, start to lift your hands off the floor one at a time, bringing your hands onto your lower back for more support.
5. Sit back on your heels and rest your hands on your thighs to center.

FULL WHEEL POSE

The full wheel pose stretches the front of your body while strengthening all down the back. It calms the brain and helps to alleviate stress and mild depression. A highly energizing pose, it stimulates the thyroid, pituitary glands, and core organs as well as improving digestion.

1 | **BEGINNER**

1 Lie on your back with the soles of your feet on the floor and your knees bent; your feet should be close to your sit bones.

2 Keep your feet hip-width apart with the outer edges of your feet parallel to the sides of the mat. Place your hands, palms down, on the floor behind your heels.

3 Squeeze your inner thighs toward one another.

4 Press into your feet and hands to push your hips up and away from the mat.

5 Press evenly into all parts of your feet.

6 Inhale to lengthen your spine; exhale to press your hips higher.

7 To come out of the pose, begin to bend your arms and legs and lower your spine one vertebra at a time to the floor.

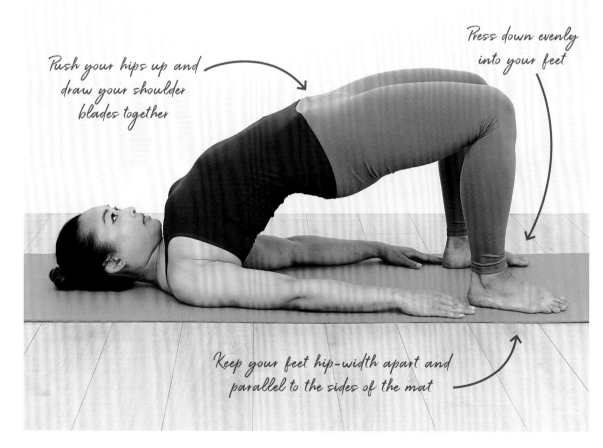

Push your hips up and draw your shoulder blades together

Press down evenly into your feet

Keep your feet hip-width apart and parallel to the sides of the mat

2 | INTERMEDIATE

Keep your legs and feet parallel

Squeeze your elbows toward one another

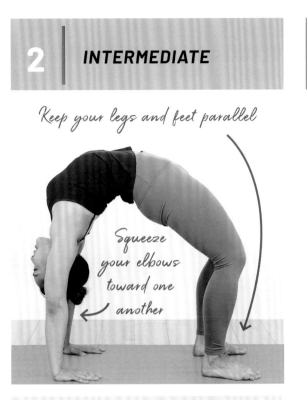

1 Begin as before.

2 Reach your arms up and overhead, and place them on the floor above your shoulders.

3 Press into your hands to lift up your shoulders, and pause with the crown of the head on the floor.

4 Press your feet down into the floor to lift your hips up to the sky, and at the same time press into your palms to lift your head.

5 Straighten your arms followed by your legs.

6 To come out of the pose, bend your elbows to bring the crown of your head to the floor, followed by the rest of your body.

7 Rest on your back with your knees bent and gently move your legs from side to side to decompress your spine and lower back.

3 | ADVANCED

Straighten your raised leg if possible

Push down into your hands and your supporting leg

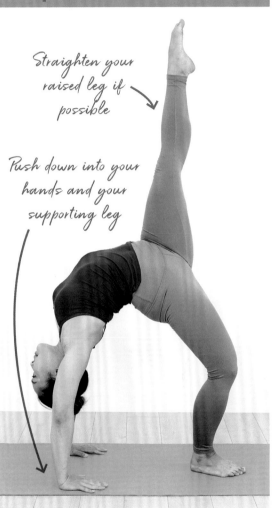

1 Begin as before. Push down into your hands and your right leg and raise your left leg up to the sky.

2 Inhale to prepare; exhale to open your shoulders. Repeat for the other leg.

3 Exit the pose as before.

DANCER POSE

The dancer pose is a combination of strength, flexibility, balance, and meditation. It strengthens the legs and core, stretches and opens the chest and shoulders, and improves balance. It also improves your ability to concentrate and focus.

1 | **BEGINNER**

1 Begin in mountain pose (*see page 26*).

2 Shift your weight onto your left leg.

3 Bend your right knee and bring your right foot up to your right glute.

4 Grab the inner arch of your right foot with your right hand, thumb facing up.

5 Lift your left arm up to the sky.

6 Lift your right leg, and at the same time bring your torso forward as a counterbalance.

7 Kick your right foot into your right hand to lift your leg higher and deepen the backbend.

8 Square your hips and draw your right hip forward and your left hip back.

9 Focus on an unmoving object for balance.

10 To come out of the pose, lower your right leg back until it is in line with your left knee. Repeat on the other side.

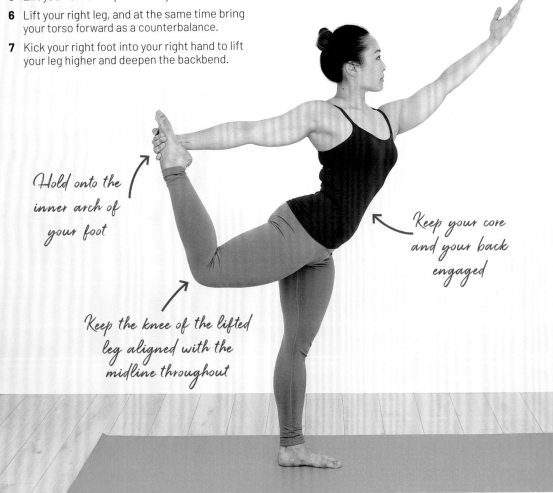

Hold onto the inner arch of your foot

Keep your core and your back engaged

Keep the knee of the lifted leg aligned with the midline throughout

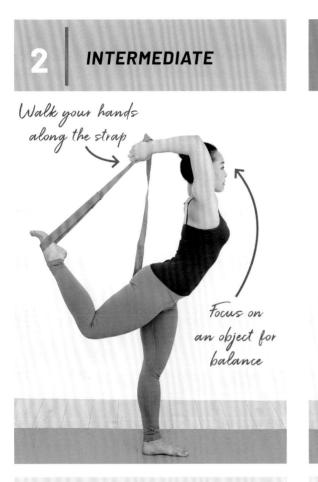

2	**INTERMEDIATE**

Walk your hands along the strap

Focus on an object for balance

3	**ADVANCED**

Press your elbows together

Press your foot into your hands

INTERMEDIATE

1   Begin as before. Hold a strap in your right hand and shift your weight onto your left leg.

2   Lift your right leg, bring your foot up behind you, and loop the strap around the top of your right foot. Pull the ends of the strap over your shoulders and lift both elbows up to the sky with your biceps by your ears.

3   Square your hips and draw your right hip forward and your left hip back.

4   Kick into the strap with your right foot, lean forward, engage your core and your back, and lift your right foot up to the sky.

5   Slowly release and repeat on the other side.

ADVANCED

1   Begin as before, with your right foot in the strap.

2   Kick into the strap and walk your hands along it toward your foot. Once you reach your foot, let go of the strap.

3   Inhale to lengthen your spine; exhale to kick back into your foot to lift your chest higher and open your shoulders farther.

4   Square your hips and draw your right hip forward and your left hip back.

5   Slowly release and repeat on the other side.

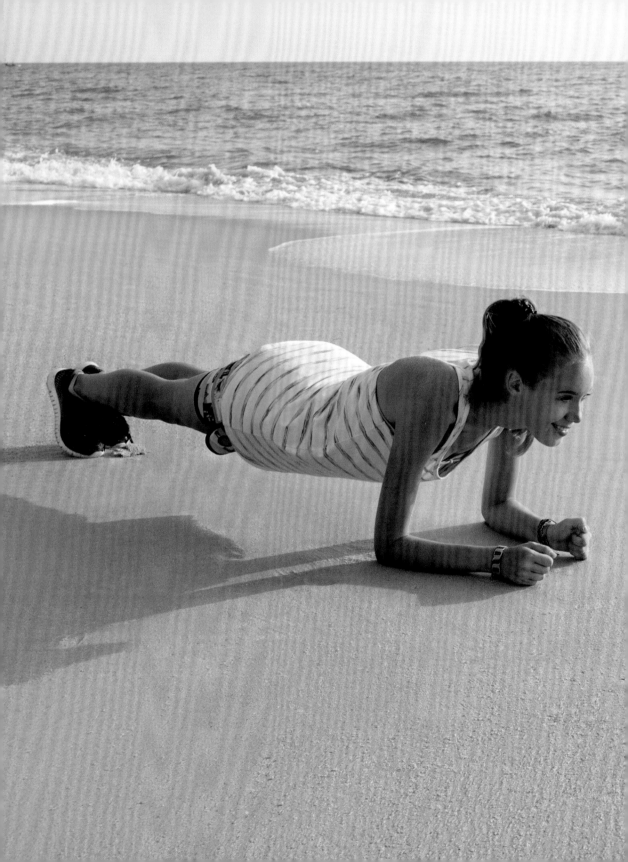

CORE STRENGTHENERS

The core is the glue that holds the whole body together.
When engaged, the core protects the back, which is crucial
in maintaining fitness over time. The poses featured here
work the solar plexus chakra, the power center of the body.
They strengthen the abdominal muscles and promote
weight loss around the midsection, boost blood circulation
throughout the internal organs, improve concentration and
balance, and help to relieve back problems by stretching
the spine and promoting better posture.

PLANK POSE

The plank pose is the cornerstone for arm balances and inversions. Always warm up your wrists and shoulders before you practice. Progress through the levels to the one-legged plank, which builds strength in the core by lifting up one leg at a time.

1 Begin on your hands and knees in table-top position (*see page 27*), with your shoulders stacked over your wrists and your hips over your knees.

2 Start to walk your knees back, coming into a flat back with your hips diagonally in line with your shoulders and knees.

3 Squeeze your knees together.

4 Draw your shoulder blades away from one another.

5 Keep your shoulders stacked over your wrists at all times.

6 Pull your belly button in and up to engage your core.

7 To come out of the pose, shift back onto your heels into child's pose (*see page 54*).

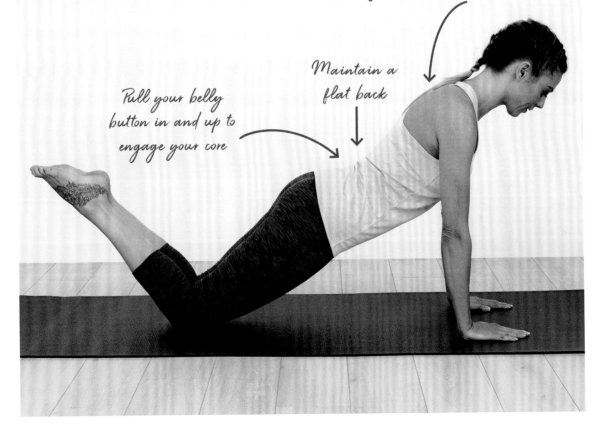

Keep your shoulders stacked over your wrists at all times

Maintain a flat back

Pull your belly button in and up to engage your core

5 Rotate your shoulders outward so your arm bones turn to face forward.

6 Elongate through the crown of your head and down through your heels.

7 On an exhale, push your hips upward and return to downward-facing dog.

1 Begin in downward-facing dog (*see pages 126–127*), with your fingers spread wide.

2 Inhale and come forward, bringing your shoulders over your wrists.

3 Lower your hips until they are diagonally in line with your shoulders and knees.

4 Draw your shoulder blades away from one another.

Squeeze your ankles together ↓

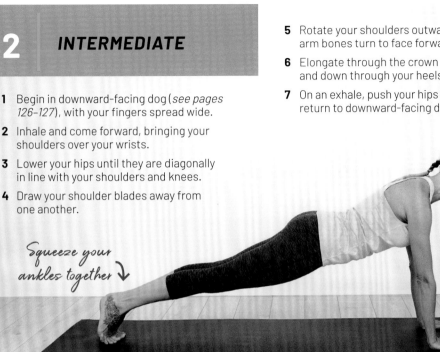

1 Come into intermediate plank pose above.

2 Squeeze into your midline, shift your weight into your left foot, and lift up your right leg, pointing the toes of your right foot; everything else stays the same.

3 Lower your right leg and return to plank pose. Repeat on the other side.

3 | **ADVANCED**

Keep your shoulders stacked over your wrists ↓

Squeeze into your midline ↘

Point your toes ↓

FOREARM PLANK

The forearm plank pose works to improve strength throughout your body—shoulders, legs, and core. It also stretches the arches of your feet, calves, hamstrings, and shoulders and is great at preparing the body for arm balances and inversions.

1 From table-top position (*see page 27*), bring your elbows to the floor underneath your shoulders.

2 Your forearms can either be parallel or, if you have tight shoulders, you can clasp your hands in a triangle.

3 Stack your shoulders over your elbows with your toes tucked under.

4 Walk your feet back one at a time until your legs are straight and your body is parallel to the floor.

5 Draw your heels toward the back of the room as you bring the crown of your head toward the front of the room.

6 Engage your quads by lifting your kneecaps.

7 Draw your tailbone down and pull your belly button in and up to engage your core.

8 Slowly come out of the pose the same way you went into it.

If you have tight shoulders, clasp your arms in a triangle

Pull your belly button in and up to engage your core

Keep your legs straight and your body parallel to the floor

1 Begin as before and come into forearm plank.

2 Engage your core, shift your weight into your left foot, and lift up your right leg, pointing the toes of your right foot.

3 Bring your right leg down and return to forearm plank pose. Repeat on the other side.

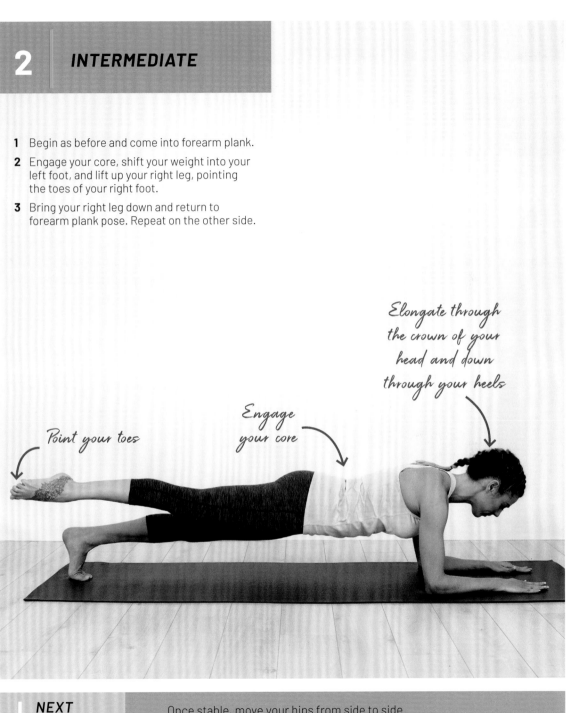

Elongate through the crown of your head and down through your heels

Engage your core

Point your toes

NEXT LEVEL Once stable, move your hips from side to side to stretch your lower back.

BOAT POSE

Creating the shape of a ship and its sails, the boat pose builds core strength as well as working the deep hip flexors. It also helps to relieve back problems by stretching the spine and improving posture, and enhances concentration and balance.

1 Begin in a sitting position with your knees bent and your feet flat on the floor.

2 Keep your spine long.

3 Lift your heels off the floor and squeeze your ankles and knees together.

4 Allow your torso to tilt back slightly, but keep your spine long and extended.

5 Use your hands to grab underneath your knees, roll your shoulders back, and draw your shoulder blades down your spine.

6 Balance on your sit bones.

7 Slowly release back to your starting position.

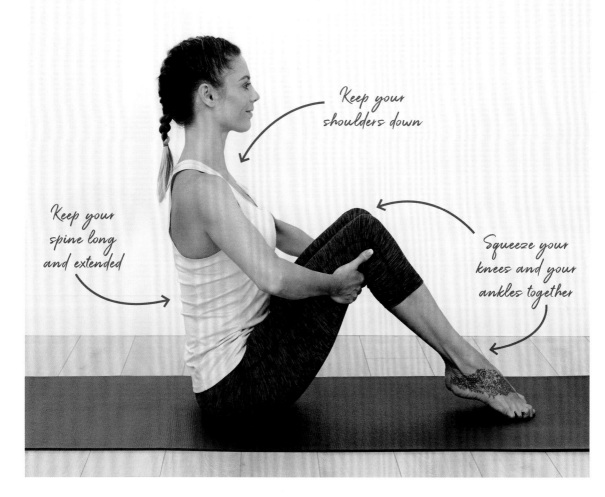

Keep your shoulders down

Keep your spine long and extended

Squeeze your knees and your ankles together

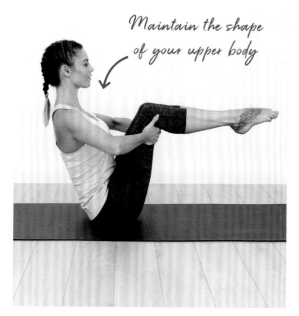

Maintain the shape of your upper body

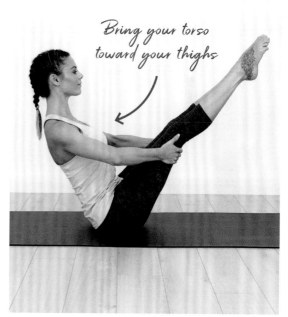

Bring your torso toward your thighs

1 Begin as before.

2 Use your hands to grab underneath your knees and slowly bend your knees so your shins are parallel to the floor without losing the shape of your upper body.

3 Roll your shoulders back and draw them down your spine.

4 Balance on your sit bones.

5 Slowly release back to your starting position.

1 Begin as before.

2 Use your hands to grab underneath your knees, then pull your knees into your chest. Bring your torso as close to your thighs as possible and begin to straighten your legs.

3 Roll your shoulders back and draw them down your spine.

4 Balance on your sit bones.

5 Slowly release back to your starting position.

CHAIR POSE

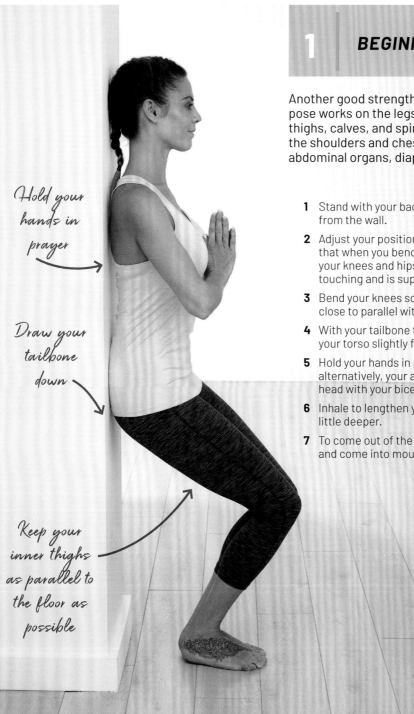

Hold your hands in prayer

Draw your tailbone down

Keep your inner thighs as parallel to the floor as possible

BEGINNER

Another good strengthening pose, the chair pose works on the legs, core, arms, ankles, thighs, calves, and spine. It also stretches the shoulders and chest and stimulates the abdominal organs, diaphragm, and heart.

1. Stand with your back a short distance away from the wall.

2. Adjust your position relative to the wall so that when you bend into chair pose, sinking your knees and hips down, your tailbone is touching and is supported by the wall.

3. Bend your knees so that your thighs are as close to parallel with the floor as possible.

4. With your tailbone touching the wall, lean your torso slightly forward over your thighs.

5. Hold your hands in prayer at the heart center; alternatively, your arms can go above your head with your biceps next to your ears.

6. Inhale to lengthen your spine; exhale to sink a little deeper.

7. To come out of the pose, straighten your legs and come into mountain pose (*see page 26*).

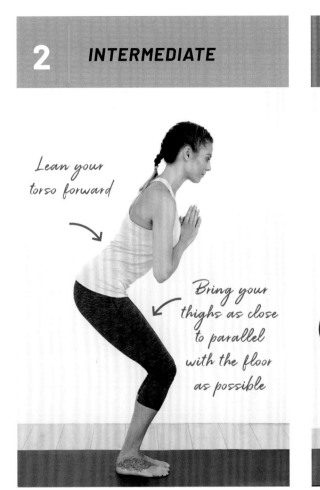

Lean your torso forward

Bring your thighs as close to parallel with the floor as possible

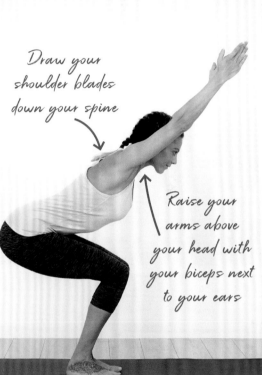

Draw your shoulder blades down your spine

Raise your arms above your head with your biceps next to your ears

1   Stand tall in mountain pose.

2   Bend your knees and lean your torso slightly forward over your thighs.

3   Your knees should be stacked over your ankles and you should be able to see your toes over your knees.

4   Draw your tailbone down.

5   Hold your hands in prayer at the heart center.

6   Inhale to lengthen your spine; exhale to sink a little deeper.

7   Come out of the pose as before.

1   Begin as before.

2   Raise your arms above your head with your biceps next to your ears and the outside edges of your hands turning toward one another.

3   Draw your shoulder blades down your spine.

4   Inhale to lengthen your spine; exhale to sink a little deeper.

5   Come out of the pose as before.

EAGLE POSE

The eagle pose strengthens and stretches the ankles, calves, thighs, hips, shoulders, and upper back. It also helps to release tightness across the shoulder blades, loosens the wrists, improves concentration and balance, and is good for joint lubrication.

1 Stand tall in mountain pose (*see page 26*).
2 Bend your knees slightly, shift your weight onto your left foot, and raise your right foot.
3 Balancing on your left foot, cross your right thigh over your left.
4 Sink a little farther into your left leg.
5 Press your forearms together in front of your face.
6 To come out of the pose, uncross your right leg back into mountain pose. Repeat on the other side.

Press your forearms together in front of your face

Cross your leg over at the thigh

Sink down into your supporting leg

2

INTERMEDIATE

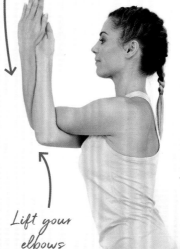

Make sure your palms are facing one another

1 Begin as before.

2 Point the toes of your right foot down toward the floor and then hook the front of your foot around behind your lower left calf (a double wrap).

3 If you are not able to double wrap, bring your toes to the floor for a kick-stand to give more support.

4 Stretch your arms forward, parallel to the floor, and spread your shoulder blades wide across the back of your torso.

5 Cross your arms in front of your torso with your left arm above your right, bend your elbows, and raise your forearms parallel to the floor with the backs of your hands facing one another.

6 Press your left hand toward the left, and your right hand toward the right, so that your palms are now facing one another.

7 Press your palms together as much as you can, lift your elbows and stretch your fingers to the sky.

8 Unwind your legs and arms to come out of eagle pose and into mountain pose. Repeat on the other side.

Draw your tailbone down

Lift your elbows

Hook the top of your foot behind the opposite calf

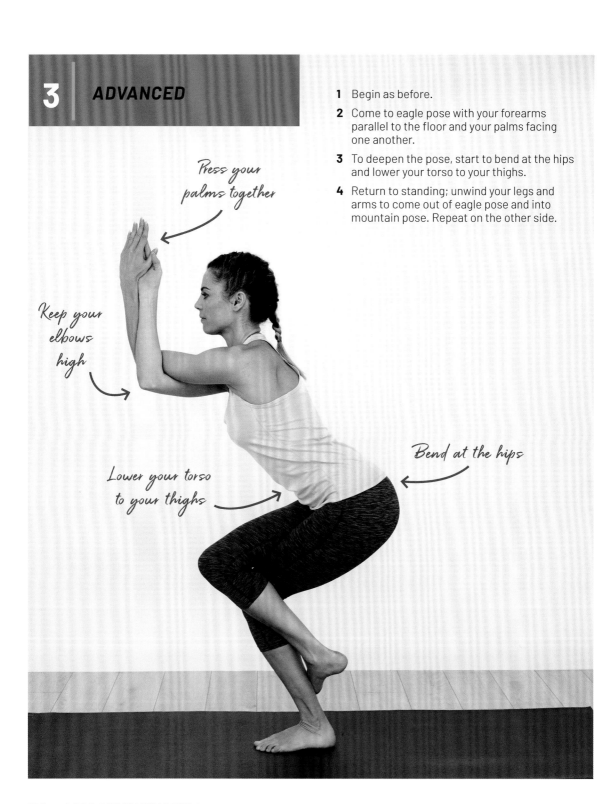

3 | *ADVANCED*

1 Begin as before.

2 Come to eagle pose with your forearms parallel to the floor and your palms facing one another.

3 To deepen the pose, start to bend at the hips and lower your torso to your thighs.

4 Return to standing; unwind your legs and arms to come out of eagle pose and into mountain pose. Repeat on the other side.

Press your palms together

Keep your elbows high

Bend at the hips

Lower your torso to your thighs

WARRIOR 3

This pose works on balance and strength, and is challenging for both the core and the entire body. It strengthens ankles and legs, tones the abs, and stretches the chest, shoulders, and hamstrings. It also improves balance and coordination.

1 Have two blocks ready at a low or high setting, whichever is the most suitable level for you.

2 Shift onto your right leg and extend your left leg straight out behind you.

3 Keep your left foot flexed and active, with your toes pointing down.

4 Square your hips and ensure they are level.

5 Draw your right kneecap up toward your hips to engage your quads and protect your knee.

6 Reach down toward the blocks with your hands and lower your torso, keeping it parallel to the floor.

7 Extend through the crown of your head and kick back with your left foot.

8 To come out of the pose, bring your left foot back to meet your right and raise your torso to a vertical position. Repeat on the other side.

Keep your torso parallel to the floor

Make sure your hips are level

Keep your foot flexed and active

Draw your kneecap up to protect your knee

1   Begin as before, this time without blocks.

2   Lower your torso, keeping it parallel to the floor, and hold your hands in prayer at the heart center.

3   Extend through the crown of your head and kick back with your left foot.

4   Hold for 5–10 breaths.

5   To come out of the pose, bring your left foot back to meet your right and raise your torso to a vertical position.

6   Repeat on the other side.

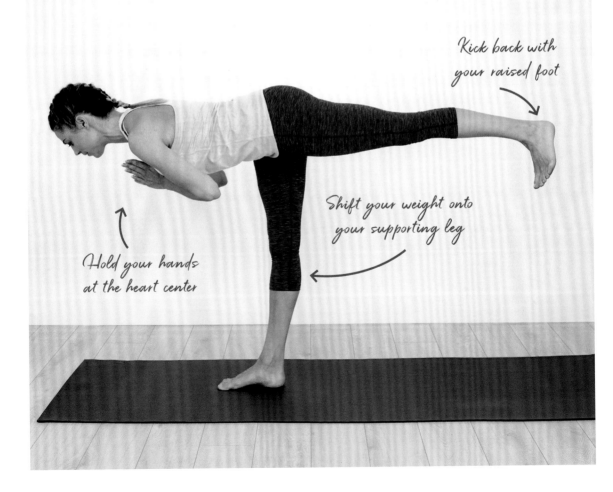

Kick back with your raised foot

Shift your weight onto your supporting leg

Hold your hands at the heart center

3 | ADVANCED

1 Begin as before.
2 Reach your arms straight out in front above your head.
3 Extend through the crown of your head and kick back with your left foot.
4 Hold for 5–10 breaths.

5 To come out of the pose, bring your left foot back to meet your right and raise your torso to a vertical position.
6 Repeat on the other side.

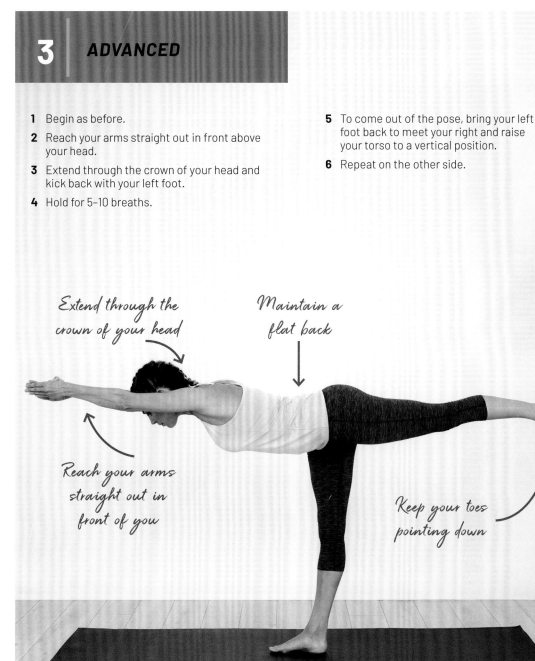

Extend through the crown of your head

Maintain a flat back

Reach your arms straight out in front of you

Keep your toes pointing down

NEXT LEVEL
For more intensity, interlace all ten fingers with your arms extended forward.

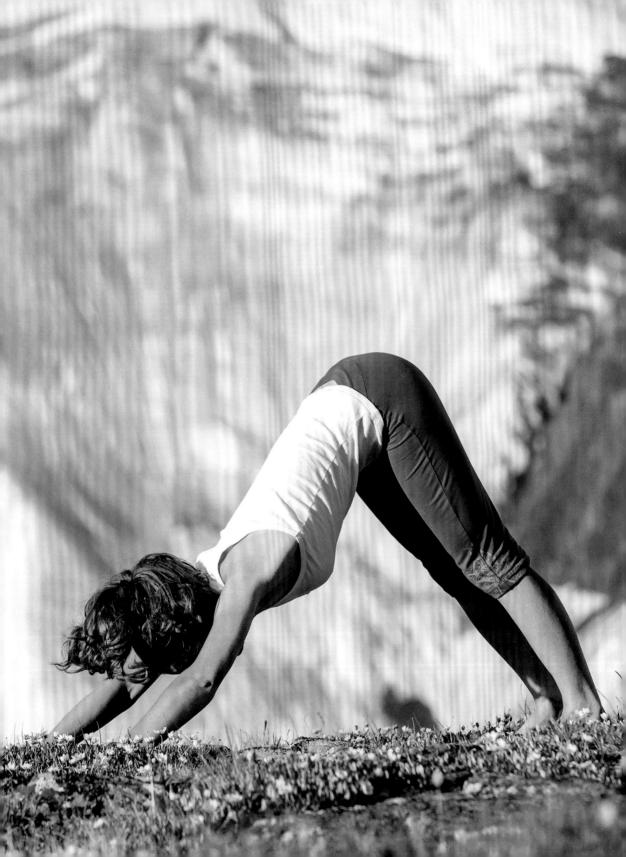

7

ARM BALANCES AND INVERSIONS

Arm balances and inversion poses both increase the flow of blood to the brain, which can have a calming effect, thereby relieving stress and anxiety. They can also shift our perspective, both literally and metaphorically, and the focus and concentration required helps us to notice our internal dialogue. Working your way toward these poses involves building strength and balance as well as confidence until you are able to let go of your fear. If you visualize yourself in the pose, your body will follow! When undertaking these poses it is important to engage your core and shoulders and to strengthen and engage your wrists and fingertips, as these will bear the entire weight of your body.

DOWNWARD-FACING DOG

In this inversion that resembles an upside-down "V" the head is below the hips. This pose helps to calm the brain, relieve stress, and improve digestion. It also energizes the body, stretches the shoulders, hamstrings, calves, arches, and hands, and strengthens the arms and legs.

1 | **BEGINNER**

1 Begin on your hands and knees in table-top position (*see page 27*), with your arms shoulder-width apart.

2 Tuck in your toes and send your hips up to the sky while opening your shoulders.

3 Draw your shoulders down and back and rotate your arms outward, keeping your elbows straight and pushing down into the first two knuckles of each hand to protect your wrists.

4 Keep your knees bent and the outer edges of your feet parallel to one another.

5 Inhale to lengthen your spine; exhale to press down into your heels and hands.

6 To come out of the pose, bring your knees back down to the floor and come into table-top position.

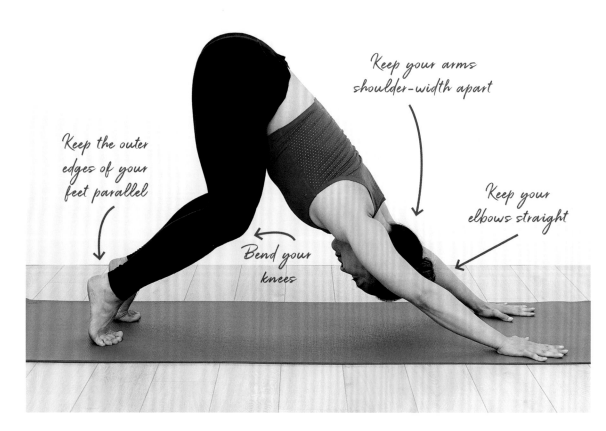

Keep your arms shoulder-width apart

Keep the outer edges of your feet parallel

Keep your elbows straight

Bend your knees

1 Begin as before, placing your hands on blocks on their lowest setting.

2 Tuck in your toes and send your hips up to the sky while opening and rotating your shoulders as before, but this time keep your knees straight, if possible.

3 Inhale to lengthen your spine; exhale to press down into your heels and hands.

4 Come out of the pose as before.

Keep your knees straight, if possible

Use your blocks on their lowest setting

1 Begin as before, this time without blocks. Keep your knees straight and your heels to the floor.

2 Inhale to lengthen your spine; exhale to press down into your heels and hands.

3 Come out of the pose as before.

3 | **ADVANCED**

Open your shoulders and rotate your arms outward

Straighten your knees and bring your heels to the floor

NEXT LEVEL

To loosen the spine, add small, dynamic movements such as pedaling the feet or shifting your weight from side to side.

DOLPHIN POSE

This pose stretches and strengthens the shoulders and helps prepare the body for future arm balances and inversions. It shares the benefits of other inversions, including relief of stress, reduced fatigue, and improved digestion.

1   From forearm plank (*see page 112*) with hands interlaced and your toes tucked in, begin to walk your feet in toward your hands.

2   Keeping your knees bent and the outer edges of your feet parallel, send your hips up to the sky and press down into your forearms to open your shoulders. Do not let your shoulders go beyond your elbows.

3   Bring the crown of your head to the floor. Keep your head in between your forearms.

4   Inhale to prepare; exhale to press into your shoulders and lift your hips up farther.

5   To come out of the pose, bring your knees to the floor and come into child's pose (*see page 54*).

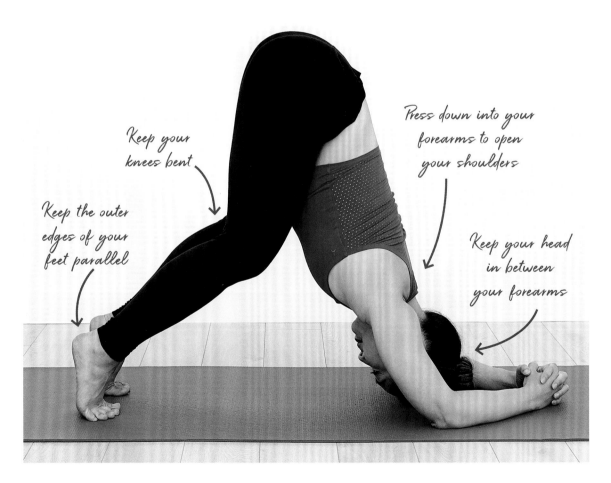

Keep your knees bent

Keep the outer edges of your feet parallel

Press down into your forearms to open your shoulders

Keep your head in between your forearms

1 Begin as before.

2 This time use straps around your forearms to stop them from splaying out. Ensure your forearms are shoulder-width apart.

3 Send your hips up to the sky; stack your hips over your shoulders and straighten your legs as much as you can.

4 Inhale to prepare; exhale to press into your shoulders and lift your hips up farther.

5 Come out of the pose as before.

Your forearms should be shoulder-width apart

Straighten your knees as much as you can

1 Begin as before, this time without straps.

2 Ensure your forearms are shoulder-width apart and engage your shoulders.

3 Straighten your knees and lower your heels to the floor.

4 Inhale to prepare; exhale to press into your shoulders and bring your heels to the floor.

5 Come out of the pose as before.

Straighten your knees

Bring your heels to the floor

CROW/CRANE POSE

This is one of the foundation arm balances—the poses that involve holding up your body weight with just your hands. The beginner position prepares you for the intermediate crow pose, while the advanced pose is the crane. It strengthens the arms, forearms, and wrists while developing core strength.

BEGINNER

1 Place a block, long side up in front of your feet.

2 With your feet shoulder-width apart come into a standing forward fold (*see page 40*) and place your hands about 12 inches in front of your feet.

3 Bend your arms and place your forehead on the block.

4 Keeping your hips lifted, lean forward and place your right knee as close to your right armpit as possible.

5 Engage your core and draw in your abs; press down into your fingertips and knuckles.

6 Inhale to prepare; exhale to lift your heel higher.

7 To come out of the pose, place both feet on the floor and press into your hands to lift your forehead away from the block. Come back into a standing forward fold with your knees bent.

Place your knee just under your armpit

Engage your core

Press your shin against the back of your upper arms

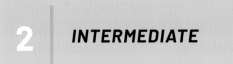

2 | INTERMEDIATE

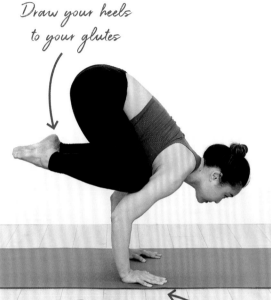

Draw your heels to your glutes

Press down into your hands for stability

1. Begin as before, this time without the block.
2. Lean forward while bending your arms; press down into your fingertips and knuckles.
3. Go up onto your toes and lift one leg, placing your knee under your armpit.
4. Do the same with the other leg, continuing to press into your hands. Pull your knees toward your armpits and round your spine.
5. Inhale to prepare; exhale to bring your heels farther toward your glutes.
6. To come out of the pose, bring both feet to the floor and come back into a standing forward fold with knees bent.

3 | ADVANCED

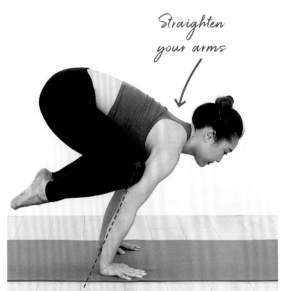

Straighten your arms

Pull your knees to your armpits

1. Begin as before.
2. Once in crow pose start to straighten your arms.
3. Engage your core and pull your knees farther up into your armpits, while drawing your heels to your glutes.
4. Inhale to prepare; exhale to bring your heels farther toward your glutes.
5. To come out of the pose, bring both feet to the floor and come back into a standing forward fold with knees bent.

SUPPORTED HEADSTAND

The headstand calms the brain and helps relieve stress while strengthening the arms, shoulders, legs, and core, and also stretches the hamstrings and the shoulders. The beginner and intermediate poses are designed to prepare you for the advanced pose—the supported headstand itself.

1 | BEGINNER

1 Come into dolphin pose (*see pages 128-129*).

2 Tuck your head in, interlace your hands, and frame your head with your elbows.

3 Inhale to prepare; exhale to stack your hips over your shoulders more.

4 To come out of the pose, bring your knees to the floor and come into child's pose (*see page 54*).

Stack your hips over your shoulders

Rest the crown of your head on the floor

Frame your head with your elbows

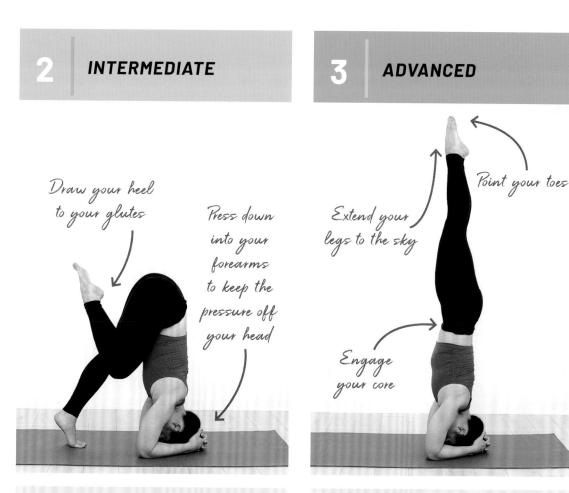

2 | INTERMEDIATE

Draw your heel to your glutes

Press down into your forearms to keep the pressure off your head

1 Begin as before.
2 Walk your feet in toward your arms.
3 Press down into your shoulders and forearms to keep the pressure off your head.
4 Bend one knee, drawing your heel to your glute.
5 Inhale to prepare; exhale to draw your heel closer to your glute.
6 Straighten your leg down to the floor and then repeat on the other side.
7 Come out of the pose as before.

3 | ADVANCED

Point your toes

Extend your legs to the sky

Engage your core

1 Begin as before.
2 Once one leg is lifted, tuck the other knee into your chest.
3 Slowly start to extend your legs straight up to the sky; do this against a wall if you're afraid of tipping over.
4 Inhale to lengthen your spine and exhale to engage your core and legs, and press down into your forearms to take the pressure off your head.
5 To come out of the pose, slowly tuck your knees into your chest, straighten one leg at a time down to the floor, and come into child's pose.

TRIPOD HEADSTAND

In a similar way to the supported headstand, this pose strengthens and stretches the body and calms the brain, helping to relieve stress. The beginner pose sets up the headstand with the crown of the head on the floor and the hands in a triangle. The intermediate pose walks the feet in and alternates lifting the legs, while the advanced pose takes you to full headstand.

1 | BEGINNER

1 Come into dolphin pose (*see pages 128-129*) and rest the crown of your head on the floor.

2 Place your hands on either side of your head about 6 inches in front. Squeeze your elbows toward one another and keep them stacked over your wrists. Raise your hips up to the sky.

3 Inhale to prepare; exhale to stack your hips over your shoulders more.

4 To come out of the pose, bring your knees to the floor and come into child's pose (*see page 54*).

Stack your hips over your elbows

Squeeze your elbows toward one another

Keep your elbows stacked over your wrists

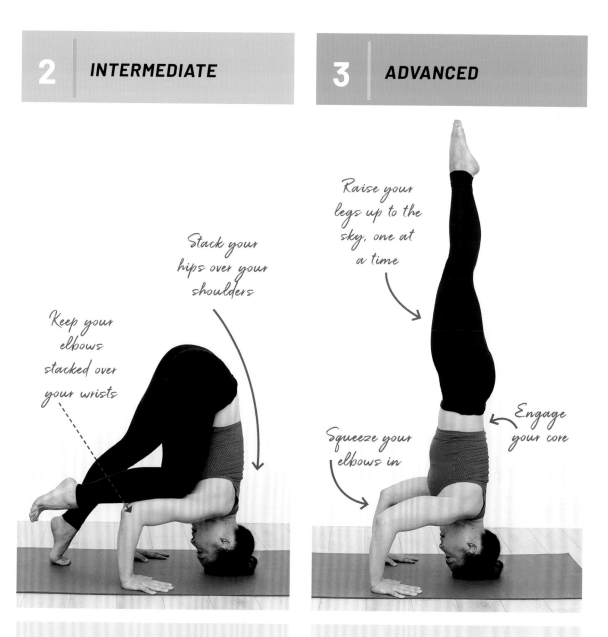

Stack your hips over your shoulders

Keep your elbows stacked over your wrists

Raise your legs up to the sky, one at a time

Engage your core

Squeeze your elbows in

1 Begin as before and walk your feet in so your hips are stacked over your shoulders. Bend one knee into your armpit.

2 Come out of the pose as before. Repeat on the other side.

1 Begin as before.

2 Engaging your core, raise each leg up to the sky.

3 Come out of the pose as before.

FOREARM BALANCE

This pose helps to increase blood flow to the brain as well as to the rest of the body and improves energy levels. It has a calming effect and can relieve stress and anxiety. It also develops upper body strength, improves balance, and increases confidence.

1 | **BEGINNER**

1 Begin in forearm plank position (*see page 112*) with your forearms parallel to one another.

2 Walk your feet up toward your hands.

3 Send your hips up to the sky while pressing down into your forearms and opening your shoulders.

4 Come into dolphin pose (*see pages 128–129*).

5 Inhale to prepare; exhale to stack your hips over your shoulders more.

6 To come out of the pose, bring your knees to the floor and come into child's pose (*see page 54*).

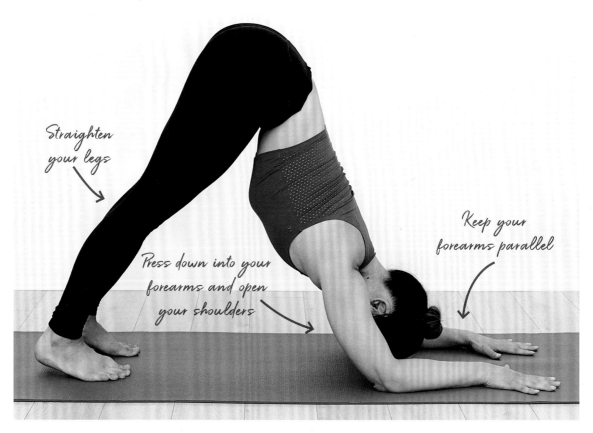

Straighten your legs

Press down into your forearms and open your shoulders

Keep your forearms parallel

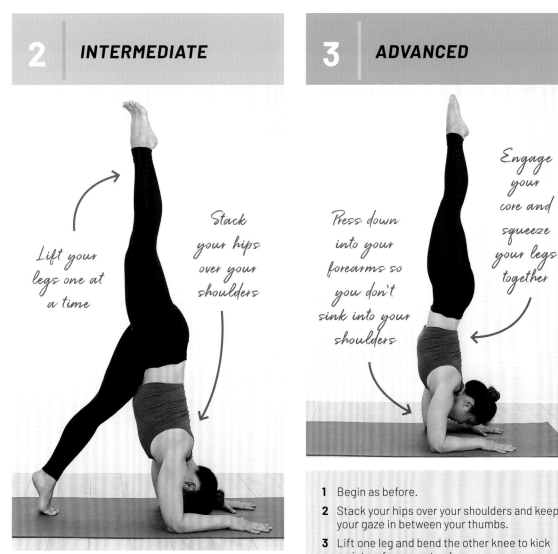

Lift your legs one at a time

Stack your hips over your shoulders

1. Begin as before.
2. Come into dolphin pose, walk your feet in toward your hands, and lift one leg straight up to the sky.
3. Inhale to prepare; exhale to come onto your toes and lift your leg higher. Repeat with the other leg.
4. Come out of the pose as before.

Engage your core and squeeze your legs together

Press down into your forearms so you don't sink into your shoulders

1. Begin as before.
2. Stack your hips over your shoulders and keep your gaze in between your thumbs.
3. Lift one leg and bend the other knee to kick up into a forearm stand.
4. Slowly bring your legs to vertical.
5. Inhale and exhale through your nose, engaging your core, glutes, and legs.
6. Lower one leg at a time to come out of the pose.
7. Practice against a wall or have a friend spot you at the hips until you are more confident.

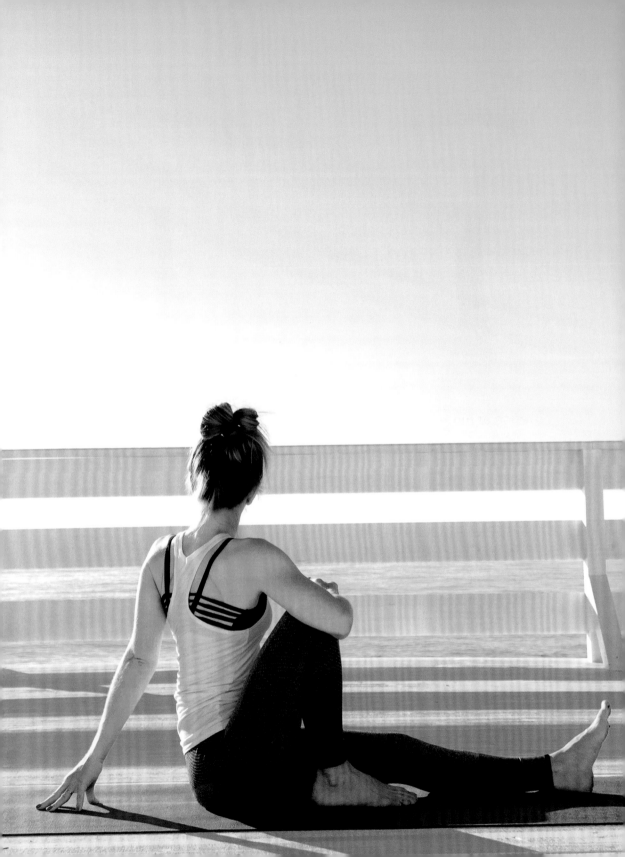

8

TWISTS

Twists rotate the spine and stretch the muscles in your back, which helps to restore and maintain the spine's natural range of motion. They can also help to alleviate lower back pain. As twists have the effect of compressing the organs in your abdominal cavity, when you release the pose the fresh circulation of blood to your organs can aid digestion and also has a detoxifying effect. Alignment is extremely important in twists for safety: make sure you inhale and lengthen the spine first, and then twist from the lower spine upward. You should avoid twists if you are pregnant or have a spinal disc injury, chronic digestive problems, or sacroiliac joint (SIJ) issues.

HALF LORD OF THE FISHES POSE

This pose energizes the spine and stretches the shoulders, hips, and neck. It also stimulates the acids and enzymes in your stomach that process the food you eat, helping you maintain a healthy metabolism and digestive system.

1   **BEGINNER**

1 Sit on the floor with your legs straight out in front of you.

2 Bend your knees, open your right hip, and place your right foot under your left leg toward the outside of your left hip.

3 Step your left foot over your right leg and prop it against the outside of your right thigh, with your left knee pointing up to the sky. Inhale.

4 Exhale and twist toward the left, pressing your left hand into the floor behind your left hip, and with your right arm around your left knee.

5 Press your left foot actively into the floor.

6 Inhale to lengthen your spine and exhale to press into the floor with your left hand and pull on your left knee with your right arm to deepen the twist.

7 Continue to twist your torso by turning toward the left.

8 Slowly release the twist and return to your starting position.

9 Repeat on the other side.

Pull on your knee to deepen the twist

Twist your torso

Press your foot into the floor

Press into the floor with your hand

2	**INTERMEDIATE**

Press your elbow against your knee and raise your hand

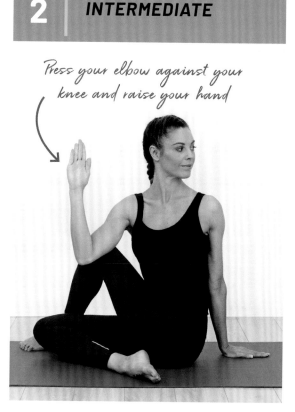

1 Begin as before.
2 On the exhale, press into the floor with your left hand and press the outside of your right elbow against the outside of your left knee.
3 Bend your right elbow and point your right hand up to the sky.
4 Continue to twist your torso by turning toward the left.
5 Slowly release the twist and return to your starting position. Repeat on the other side.

3	**ADVANCED**

Reach one arm under your knee

Reach the other arm behind your back

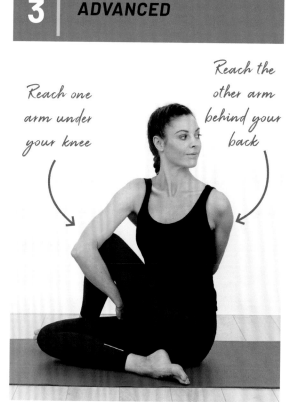

1 Begin as before.
2 To go for the bind, bring the upper right arm to the outside of the upper left thigh.
3 With your torso snug against your thigh, work your right upper arm farther onto your left leg until the back of your shoulder presses against your knee.
4 Start to reach under your left knee with your right hand and reach your left arm around your lower back to link your hands together for a bind, hooking your fingers together.
5 Slowly release the twist and return to your starting position. Repeat on the other side.

RECLINED SUPINE TWIST

The reclined supine twist pose is a therapeutic yoga posture that stretches the back muscles and glutes, massages the back and hips, lengthens and decompresses the spine, and encourages a flow of fresh blood to the digestive organs. It is beneficial immediately after practicing backbends to realign the spine.

| 1 | **BEGINNER** |

1 Lie on your back.

2 Bend your knees into your chest with your arms wrapped around your shins.

3 Hold onto your knees with your hands.

4 Shift your hips slightly to the left.

5 Slowly guide your knees to the right side of your body, engaging your core on the descent.

6 Turn your head to the left.

7 Stretch your arms straight out to the sides from your shoulders to create a T-shape.

8 Relax your shoulders away from your ears.

9 Slowly come back to the center, bringing both knees into your chest. Repeat on the other side.

Turn your head in the opposite direction to your knees

Relax your shoulders away from your ears

Engage your core as you lower your legs

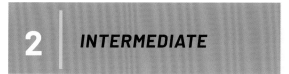

2 | INTERMEDIATE

1 Lie on your back with your legs stretched out.
2 Draw your left knee into your chest.

3 Shift your hips slightly to the left.
4 Take your left knee with your right hand and guide it over to the right side of your body.
5 Turn your head to the left to deepen the twist.
6 Stretch your left arm out to the side.
7 Slowly come back to the center, bringing both knees into your chest. Repeat on the other side.

Stretch your arm out to the side

Guide your knee over to the opposite side

3 | ADVANCED

1 Begin as before.
2 Draw your left knee into your chest and wrap your left leg over your right thigh, double wrapping if possible.

3 Take your left knee with your right hand and guide it over to the right side of your body.
4 Bend your arms at the elbows and stretch them above your head to open your chest even farther.
5 Slowly come back to the center, bringing both knees into your chest. Repeat on the other side.

Turn your head to deepen the twist

Double wrap your legs

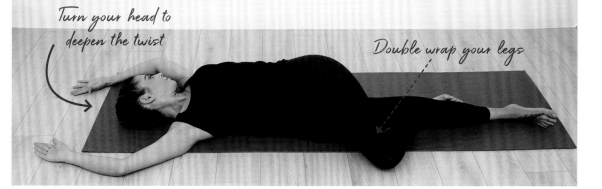

TWISTED MONKEY LUNGE

The twisted monkey lunge or crooked monkey pose is great for athletes as it works hips, quads, glutes, and hip flexors. The twist stretches the whole length of the spine and massages the internal organs, aiding digestion and improving circulation.

1 **BEGINNER**

1 Come into a low lunge with your right foot forward and your right knee stacked directly over your right ankle.

2 Stack your left heel over your toes with your weight on the ball of your left foot.

3 Place your left arm on the floor and lift your right arm up to the sky by your ear.

4 Turn your right shoulder back and your torso to the right as you begin to turn your hips, coming up onto the outside of your left foot.

5 Sweep your right arm behind you so it is parallel to the floor. Turn your gaze to your arm.

6 To come out of the pose, bring your right hand down to the floor beside your left and twist your torso back to the front. Bring your left knee to the floor, step your right knee back, and come into table-top position (*see page 27*). Repeat on the other side.

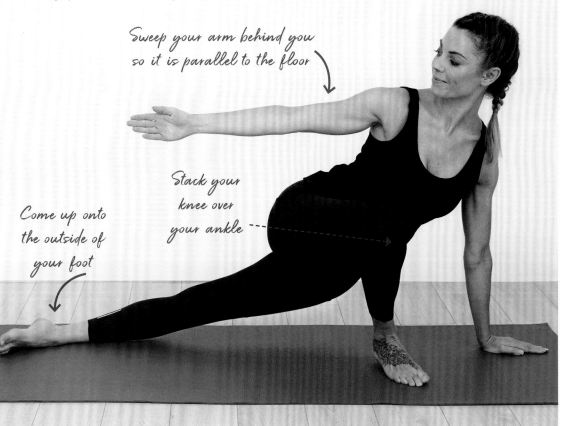

Sweep your arm behind you so it is parallel to the floor

Stack your knee over your ankle

Come up onto the outside of your foot

1 Come into a low lunge with your right foot forward and your left knee on the floor.

2 Place your left hand on the floor.

3 Holding both ends of the strap in your right hand, bend your left knee and hook the strap around your left foot.

4 Inhale to lengthen your spine; exhale to twist a little deeper.

5 Your right foot can turn out slightly together with your right knee.

6 To come out of the pose, release the strap and bring your left leg down to the floor. Bring your right hand down to the floor beside your left and come into a table-top position. Repeat on the other side.

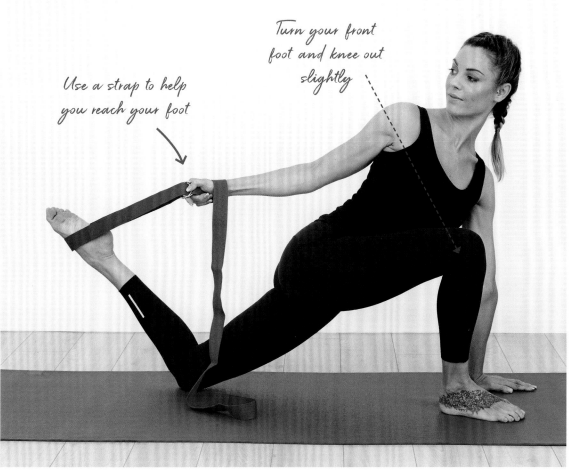

Turn your front foot and knee out slightly

Use a strap to help you reach your foot

1 Begin as before.

2 Bend your left knee and reach back with your right arm to grab the outside of your foot or ankle.

3 Slowly drop your left forearm to the floor.

4 Inhale to lengthen your spine; exhale to twist a little deeper.

5 Open your chest up to the sky.

6 To come out of the pose, release your left foot slowly and straighten your left leg down to the floor. Bring your right arm next to your left forearm, step your right knee back, and come into table-top position. Repeat on the other side.

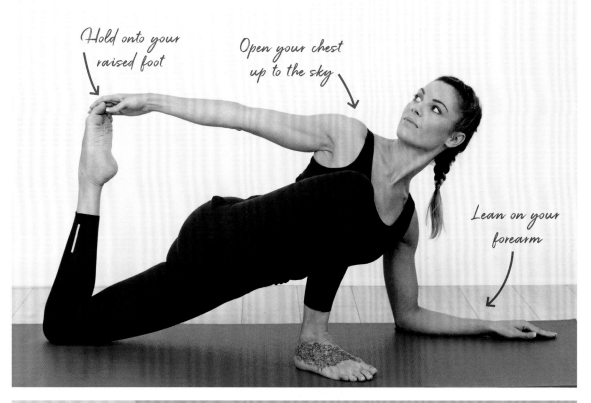

Hold onto your raised foot

Open your chest up to the sky

Lean on your forearm

NEXT LEVEL   To deepen the stretch, draw your back heel in toward your glute.

REVOLVED CRESCENT LUNGE

The revolved crescent lunge pose creates stability throughout your entire body. As with other twists it strengthens and stretches the spine, hips, legs, and glutes. It also stimulates and detoxifies the internal organs and aids in improving digestion and boosting metabolism.

1 Come into a low lunge with your right foot forward and your left knee on the floor.

2 Stack your right knee over your right ankle and ensure your left leg is parallel with the sides of the mat.

3 Take a block in your left hand and place it on the inside or outside (to go deeper) of your right foot at a low or high setting, whichever is the most suitable level for you.

4 Plant your left hand on the block; if it is outside your right foot, hook your arm over the outside of your right thigh.

5 Reach your right arm up to the sky.

6 Inhale to lengthen your spine; exhale and twist your body to the right.

7 Lift your chest up to the sky.

8 Slowly come out of the twist. Repeat on the other side.

Lift your arm to the sky and look up at your hand

Place the block outside your foot to go deeper

Make sure your back leg is parallel with the sides of the mat

1. Begin as before.

2. Frame your right foot with your hands.

3. Tuck in the toes of your left foot and lift your left knee off the floor, stacking your right knee over your right ankle, and your left heel directly over your toes.

4. Inhale and bring your arms up to the sky for a crescent lunge (*see pages 69–71*).

5. Exhale and bring your hands to the heart center as you twist to the right, hooking the outside of your left elbow over the outside of your right thigh.

6. Bring your chest to your hands.

7. Inhale to lengthen your spine; exhale to twist a little deeper.

8. Press your hands together and push against them to deepen the twist farther. Aim to get the back of your left shoulder against the outside of your right knee.

9. Slowly come out of the twist.

10. Repeat on the other side.

2 | INTERMEDIATE

Press your hands together at the heart center

Keep your heel stacked over your toes

Stack your knee over your ankle

1. Begin as before.

2. To go for the bind, bring your upper left arm to the outside of your upper right thigh.

3. With your torso snug against your thigh, work your left upper arm farther down onto your outer leg as far as you can. Aim to get the back of your shoulder against your knee.

4. Start to reach under your right knee with your left hand and bring your right arm around your lower back to link your hands together for a bind, hooking your fingers together.

5. Inhale to lengthen your spine; exhale to twist a little deeper.

6. Continue to twist your chest up to the sky.

7. To come out of the pose, let go of your hands and slowly come out of the twist.

8. Repeat on the other side.

3 | ADVANCED

Twist your chest up to the sky

Link your hands together to make a bind

Keep your torso snug against your thigh

REVOLVED TRIANGLE POSE

The revolved triangle pose strengthens and stretches the legs, hips, and spine, opens the chest, and helps to improve breathing. It also relieves mild back pain and stimulates the abdominal organs.

1 Begin in mountain pose (*see page 26*).

2 Bring your right leg forward about 3-4ft and turn your left foot out to 90 degrees.

3 Take a block with your left hand and place it on the inside or outside (to go deeper) of your right foot at a low or high setting, whichever is the most suitable level for you.

4 Square your hips to the front and draw your left hip forward and your right hip back.

5 Inhale and lift both arms; exhale and reach your left arm forward and your right arm back, coming into a standing twist.

6 Lower your left arm down to the block.

7 Reach your right arm up to the sky.

8 Inhale to lengthen your spine; exhale to twist a little deeper.

9 Look up toward your left hand.

10 To come out of the pose, engage your core to lift your left hand off the block and come back to standing. Repeat on the other side.

Look up toward your raised arm

Rest your lower hand on the block

Turn your back foot to 90 degrees

1. Begin as before, this time without the block.
2. Slowly lower your left hand down to the floor on the inside or outside of your right foot.
3. Reach your right arm up to the sky.
4. Inhale to lengthen your spine; exhale to twist a little deeper.
5. Look up toward your right hand.
6. Come out of the pose as before.
7. Repeat on the other side.

2 | INTERMEDIATE

Keep your arms in line

Make sure your hips are square

Keep your legs straight

Reach your hand down to the floor, either inside or outside your front foot

1 Begin as before.

2 To go for the bind, bring your left upper arm farther onto your right outer leg until the back of your shoulder presses against your right knee.

3 Start to reach under your right knee with your left hand, and reach your right arm around your lower back to link your hands together for a bind, hooking your fingers together.

4 Inhale to lengthen your spine; exhale to twist a little deeper.

5 To come out of the pose, let go of the bind, engage your core, and come back to standing. Repeat on the other side.

3 | **ADVANCED**

Link your hands for a bind, hooking your fingers together

Reach the other arm behind your lower back

Reach one arm around behind your knee

Continue to twist your chest upward

REVOLVED HALF-MOON POSE

The revolved half-moon pose combines the challenge of balancing with the detoxifying benefits of a twist. It builds stability in the core muscles and helps to develop physical and mental stamina.

1 BEGINNER

1 Begin by standing with your right foot forward and your left foot back.

2 Take one or more blocks and place about 1ft in front of your right leg, slightly to the left. Use a low or high setting.

3 Push down into your right foot.

4 Inhale and lean forward, placing your left hand on the block(s), while lifting your left leg straight back.

5 Flex the toes of your left foot toward the floor, with your foot pointing straight down.

6 Inhale to lengthen your spine; exhale and twist your torso to the right, lifting your right arm up to the sky.

7 Bring the crown of your head forward and kick back into your left foot.

8 Square your hips, lowering your left hip in line with your right.

9 To come out of the pose, bend your right knee and engage your core to lift your left hand off the block(s). Bring your left leg down to the floor and come back to standing. Repeat on the other side.

Elongate your spine

Look up toward your raised arm

Point the outside of your back foot straight down to the floor

1 Begin as before.

2 Fix your gaze about 1ft in front of your right leg.

3 Push down into your right foot.

4 Inhale and lean forward, placing your left hand on the floor, while lifting your left leg straight back.

5 Flex the toes of your left foot toward the floor, with the outside of the foot pointing straight down.

6 Inhale to lengthen your spine.

7 Exhale and twist your torso to the right, lifting your right arm up to the sky.

8 Bring the crown of your head forward and kick back into your left foot.

9 Square your hips, lowering your left hip in line with your right.

10 Come out of the pose as before. Repeat on the other side.

Make sure your hips are square

Flex your toes

Push your weight into your supporting foot

Place your hand on the floor

1 Begin as before.

2 Start to bend your left leg, bringing your left heel to your left glute.

3 Reach back with your right hand to catch your left foot or ankle.

4 Inhale to lengthen your spine.

5 Exhale and twist your torso to the right.

6 Push into your hand to lift your chest and open your shoulders even farther.

7 To come out of the pose, release your left foot slowly and straighten your left leg down to the floor. Bend your right knee and engage your core to lift your left hand off the floor and come back to standing. Repeat on the other side.

Reach back to catch your foot

Bring your raised heel to your glute

Push into your hand to lift your chest and open your shoulders

"Flexibility begins in the mind; it takes time and through consistent practice, breath, and positive thinking, you'll get there. The end goal isn't to be the most flexible person in the world but it's about your journey through breath and movement to gain a better understanding and connection with your mind and body. Be patient with yourself and know that all is coming."

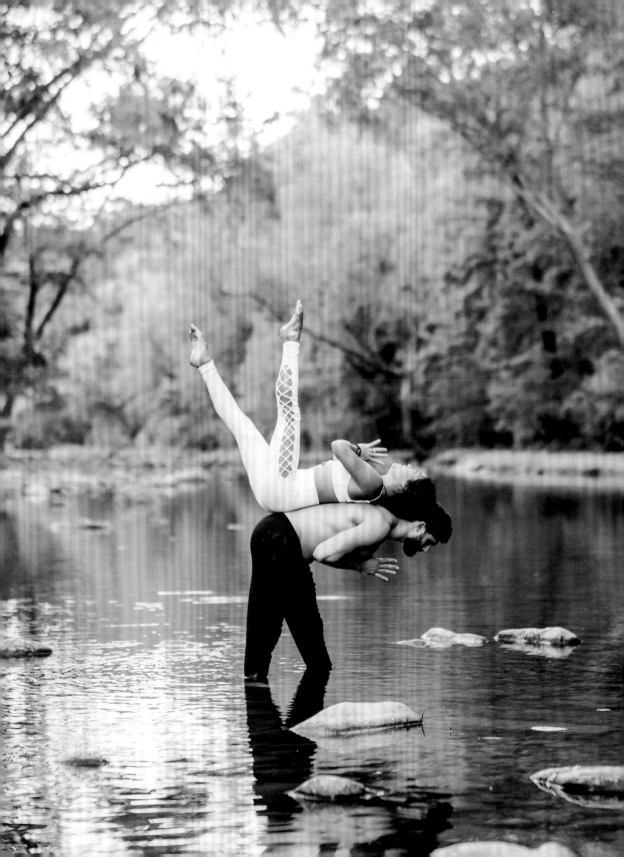

INDEX

PICTURE CREDITS

Photographs by Ruth Jenkinson, except the following: pages 4–5 Photo by Jordan Siemens/Taxi via Getty Images; page 12 Rebecca Gibson (@bowlingandyoga); page 13 Shaeeda Sween (@westindianbella); pages 14–15 Erica Ippolito (@miss___erica); page 16 Yoga Vared (@yogavered); page 17 Joe Lizz (@Joe_lizzzzzz_yoga); pages 7, 8, 11, 157 and 160 Max and Liz Lowenstein; Shutterstock, Inc: pages 18 Iam_Anupong; 36–37 MS Mikel; 38, 64, 124 My Good Images; 52 Maryna Pleshkun; 92 icsnaps; 108 Chemomorova Olesia; 138 Yolya Ilyasova

ACKNOWLEDGMENTS

Photographer: Ruth Jenkinson
Models: Charles Ruhmund, Ella Durston/Source Models; Wen Dai
Designer: Lucy Palmer
Copy editor: Katie Hewett
Proofreader: Jane Donovan
Indexer: Christine Shuttleworth
Production: Gary Hayes

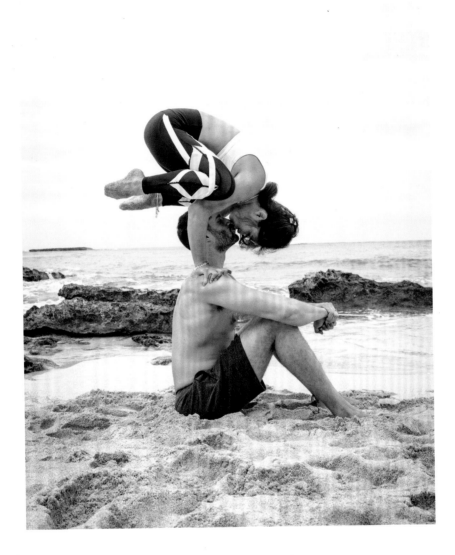

"To our teachers and their teachers,
may we disseminate the knowledge to
future generations as best as we can."